How to Flirt with Men

The Complete Dating Guide for Women Who Want to Seduce a Man, Make Him Chase You, and Keep Your Man Interested

Table of Contents

Introduction

Worldwide culture tends to put women at a disadvantage when it comes to dating. A woman can see a man she desires but can't openly make the first move for fear of being labeled cheap or desperate. Thousands of years of this type of societal conditioning has subdued women to settle for unhappy relationships while they watch helplessly as their ideal man chases after other women completely oblivious of them. But the times and tides are changing. Women are no longer waiting patiently for the man they want. They are cleverly utilizing their powerful innate abilities to build the type of relationships they want.

Unfortunately, not all women know how to do this and it is not your fault if you fall into this category. While a few women have mastered the art of attracting the men they want, a large number of us—mostly good girls—still don't know why all the good men are taken by the seemingly bad girls! But the good news is that you can now learn exactly how to stack the dating odds in your favor by learning and using the techniques in this book.

This book is specifically written to teach women how to flirt. You will learn practical ways to attract men using different techniques that are designed to pique men's interest in you. This book teaches you the proper way to utilize your inner charm on any man to get him hooked. Whether you are trying to capture the heart of your ideal man for keeps or you are only interested in flings, you'll find a tone of useful information in this amazing book. The powerful "retention tools" shared in this book will help you to create the type of relationships that you desire and deserve. But beyond just starting a relationship, you will also learn how to keep the flames of your relationship aglow even after a very long time.

This is not a book of theories, so be ready to apply what you are about to learn. The methods I share in this book are time-tested techniques gathered from the experiences of countless women over several years. They work, but you must be willing to put them into practice.

Whether you are shy like many other women or you are the outgoing type, you will be delighted to discover the fun-filled game of flirting that can change your entire adult life. But as with any other game, there are rules that must be followed to score points. If you are not willing to play by the rules, I'm afraid you will not get the results you seek. You are probably better off seeking other forms of dating and relationship solutions. What is contained here will only be of benefit to the woman who is willing to abide by the flirting rules which, by the way, are very simple to follow.

Although this book is written for women seeking to improve their dating skills, it is particularly targeted at women between the ages of 20 to 40 years. Older women may find that their perspective about dating, love, and life in general may have significantly shifted from how it used to be when they were younger and may not find the ideas in this book particularly applicable to them. But this is not to say older women cannot date any man of their choosing using these techniques.

I invite you, my fellow woman, to study this book with an open mind. I ask that you temporarily suspend whatever beliefs and notions you may hold about flirting and put aside any fears or worries that you may have about men and dating.

Here's to your success as you learn how to flirt and seduce the man of your dreams!

Chapter 1

Understanding Flirting

As ladies, we get a kick from knowing that a man is dying to be with us, to spend time with us, and to share intimate moments with us. We love it! But we don't all know exactly how to make men *feel* this way about us. Notice that I didn't say we don't know how to make men *think* this way. Men generally would think flirtingly about almost any woman if they want to—men are hardwired that way. But to get a man to feel helplessly drawn to you takes some extra skills. If you are lucky, a man can be strongly attracted to you without any conscious effort on your part. I say lucky because these days it takes quite a bit of deliberate effort to get men chasing after you. With the increasing number of ladies looking like picture-perfect sex goddesses, it is somewhat difficult to get and hold the attention of an average modern man without doing something extra.

Getting a guy's attention is pretty simple if you know how to go about it. Sex and sex appeal—anything that reminds a man of sex—can hold a guy's attention. But as simple as this may sound, you can get it all wrong and push men away from you. So, in this chapter, I'm going to outline some simple and basic rules of getting a guy's attention (and don't mind my usage of "guy" and "man." I use them interchangeably because, to me, they basically mean the same thing).

But before you proceed, I'll like to give a little warning. The flirting and seduction techniques in this book are effective. I strongly suggest that you take some time to find out the relationship status of the man you want to attract. They may already be married, attached, off-limits, or taken. I do not intend for this book to make you cause pain to another woman. My goal for writing this book is to help women all over the world who are having a difficult time embracing and expressing their feminine power to bring them the happy relationship they desire and deserve.

Charm, Flirting, Seduction: What Do You Really Want?

I see a lot of women (young and old) who feel very frustrated because the men they are desperately trying to get and keep end up being their "good friends" or confidants rather than passionately chasing after them. It is no surprise that many women find themselves in this situation; our upbringing contributes a lot to this. Many women were raised to believe good girls are not flirtatious. And who doesn't want to be a good girl? But the problem with that is good girls are more likely to become good friends than their bad girl counterparts. The so-called bad girls have the odds in their favor when it comes to getting the attention of the man they desire and even the ones they don't like.

The frustration stems from the fact that many women are in a game that they just can't win because of the ideas they have about the game itself. Using an outmoded rule book—something that worked for women centuries ago—and expecting to get the result of the modern-day woman is unrealistic. But what could you possibly be doing wrong that is turning you into a friend instead of a potential lover—a treasure to be passionately desired? And how can you change all of that? To know what you are likely doing wrong and how to change it, you need to first understand the difference between the art of being charming, flirtatious, and seductive. Confusing these three or using them wrong is probably one of the biggest reasons a man would think of a woman as his good friend instead of someone he passionately desires to be with.

Charm

To be charming is to possess the personal quality of being delightful or fascinating. As a charming lady, you have some good measure of personal attractiveness that makes you influence others to like you. People love being around a charming person because charming people combine humor and good manners. To put it very simply, to be charming is the quality of making others feel good when they are with you.

To be charming is the first step to being likable and that is where the mistake for many ladies starts and ends. If you are thinking that being charming alone can get you the man you want, well, you may be in for a long time of frustration. I am not suggesting that men don't like charming ladies; they do, but it takes more than being charming to get a man to really want to be with you. Again, you can be lucky and find a man that is contented with charming alone, but such men are generally few and far between.

The problem with being charming is that, by itself, being charming is not inherently sexual. You can be charming to your boss, your brother, your neighbor, or even your grandmother. It is a quality that is expected of every sociable person, male and female alike. Being charming is a quality that every woman who wants to have men interested in her should possess, but it alone doesn't get the job done satisfactorily. Charm has to be combined with other qualities (flirtatiousness and seductiveness) to make a man go beyond noticing and liking your personality. Having a combination of these qualities makes you a charming lady who possesses a strong sexual appeal. It is the sexual appeal part of the equation that makes a man want to chase after you.

Charm alone is likely to remind a man of his mother, sister, or a good friend. And if that is the only quality you possess as a woman, then you are very likely to become a man's trusted ally and not his desire. The hunter in a man wants more than a charming lady. This is why many married men love their wives but still chase after other women. If you have the intention of getting a man insanely interested in you even after being with him for a long time, you will need to up your game from being only charming to being flirty and seductive as well. We'll cover how to use these powerful "retention tools" (as I like to call them) in this book.

To be clear, being a charming woman is not a bad thing at all. In fact, it is a prerequisite to being powerfully attractive and irresistible. Trying to flirt with a man without possessing a charming quality will make a man think of you as being creepy. And trying to be seductive without charm makes you appear very desperate and pathetic—both are a huge turn-off for men. A flirty and seductive behavior devoid of charm is what people usually count as sexual harassment. The basic ingredient—charm—that would have made the moves sexually appealing is lacking.

Flirting

Although the phrase "plausible deniability," is often associated with the military, politics, business and espionage, it is the best phrase I can find to describe the benefit of being flirty especially for a lady. I don't want to go into the details of how our society has conditioned women to wait for men to chase after them and why a woman is looked down upon if she dares to approach a man. However, times are changing and women are beginning to "take matters into their hands." But to preserve her dignity, a woman should be able to deny that she made the first move. This is where flirting comes in handy.

Generally, to be flirtatious means to behave or act in a playfully sexual way to attract another person. Although it has a sexual connotation, flirting doesn't openly confirm sexual intention. This is why a lady can flirt with a man and easily deny (with a straight face, I might add) ever having any sexual intent. Smiling at a guy, for example, or even saying something like, "I like the beautiful look in your eyes," doesn't necessarily mean you want to have sex or start a relationship with him. However, it gives him something to think about. Usually, flirting is light, humorous and even innocent, yet it can be used to plant suggestive thoughts in the minds of any man. If you are already charming and you plant suggestive thoughts in the mind of a guy, you are setting the stage for his hunter instinct to get to work.

Flirting is used in a comparatively limited context than charm. While a lady can be charming to almost anyone, it is not appropriate to flirt with certain people and in certain places. For example, flirting with your boss in the office may not be a very good idea. Flirting with a married man may or may not be appropriate depending on your personal beliefs and what your intentions are. In any case, for this tool to have the intended effect, you need to first be a charming woman or else you'll be sending the wrong signals to a man. In subsequent sections and chapters, I shall go into the details on how to flirt; the proper use of flirting techniques and tricks that will make you appear innocent even when you are caught flirting red-handed. Also, if you do not want to appear overly expressive, stick with charming and flirting. However, if you want to take your game to an entirely different level, I'll suggest that you consider learning and perfecting the art of seduction.

Seduction

In chapter 4, I'll discuss the art of seduction. Please don't jump to that chapter just yet. Patience is necessary to understand how to apply these powerful tools. Let's take things one at a time, shall we? Great!

To a lot of women, to be seductive means to come on to a man aggressively. Doing this usually makes you look like an ignorant fool to a man and shows your lack of charm. Unless you share a very intimate relationship with a man, try not to be too forward in your seductiveness. Whatever you do, remember that you are a lady and not just some cheap hooker on the street. People tend to have the wrong notion that being seductive means being cheap or lowbrow, but that is very far from being correct.

Seduction, as used in this book, means *skillfully* enticing someone with your words and actions in ways that can result in sexual activities. The word to keep in mind is "skillfully." When done improperly, it can send the wrong signal to the man you are trying to attract or seduce. But when done right, seduction can be the number one temptation your dream man will find difficult to resist.

To skillfully put seduction to good use, always remember that:

- It has to be slow, deliberate, and very tempting. The slower and more deliberate you are, the more the man thinks you are in control. This will increase the value he has for you, and he will go all out to hunt you down. Men generally don't place a high value on a woman they got cheaply.

- It is not obviously aggressive. You don't need to do a lot of persuasion and convincing to get a man to do what you want if you have seduced him. If you have to put in extra effort to convince him, it shows he's not interested in your proposal and you should give it a rest. If you are trying to seduce a man into having sex with you, for example, and it is beginning to take too much convincing, let him go. Continuing may leave you with a seriously bruised ego or even a sexual harassment suit.

- Seduction is sexy and subtle. Touching can sometimes be necessary, but it is not required. A seductive whisper in the ear, a knowing wink, and a slow deliberate crossing or un-crossing of your legs are all sexy and subtle moves that can leave a lasting impression on a man than grabbing his crotch.

- It has to be classy with a sexual appeal. There is really no need for verbally or visually detailing body parts in a bid to seduce a man. That's not classy at all. Instead, be gentle and use euphemisms. For example, instead of sexting a man, say things like, "Would you like to see my etchings?" Being too literal can be a turn off for men and make you appear less ladylike.

The Irresistible Woman

Here's a little something for you to try. Open your browser and search for "the irresistible woman." You'll find links to several articles listing 5, 8, 10, or even 18 qualities that make a woman irresistible. But the truth is, some women don't have as nearly as half of these qualities, yet men find them very irresistible. It doesn't matter whether you have the features of a model or not; it certainly doesn't matter whether or not you are goal-driven, highly intelligent, humble, or exceptionally smart. These things are good and can get you far in your career and other areas of life, but may not be exactly what you need to attract and keep a man. What matters is knowing how to use your innate feminine energy to create and maintain attraction long enough to get a man to like you. You can achieve that by combining your inner charm with flirting and being seductive. Any other quality you possess—confidence, honesty, ability to nurture, or being self-directed—are the spices that can keep a relationship going after you have established it.

A woman who knows the difference between charming, flirting and seduction, and also knows how and when to use these powerful tools is an irresistible woman. She can have any man she desires because she knows what makes men tick. This is the type of woman this book is intended to make you into by the time you finish reading and applying the suggestions. If you do not want men to flock around you, kindly ignore the suggestions in this book, or better still, stop reading at this point. But I know you're reading this book because you want to be the cynosure of not just any man but the ideal man or men you desire. Yes! You can make any number of men irresistibly chase after you and have all the fun you truly desire and deserve. But first, let us understand the game of flirting.

Flirting: The Game

Flirting is a game—the type of game where you can convey your interest to someone (in this case a man) while skillfully avoiding possible embarrassment. The type of flirting I discuss in this book is aimed at establishing a sexual or romantic encounter with any man you desire. If you play the game right, you can create a spark in any man and keep it burning for as long as you want. You can also put out the spark as quickly as you choose, especially if you are only interested in a casual relationship and not a long-term, committed relationship.

Essentially, flirting has three different levels and intensities, namely, public, social and private flirting.

Public Flirting

Any woman can do this because it is usually amusing, spontaneous, and innocent with the goal of simply making someone feel good about themselves or their day. In fact, many people do this without knowing that they are flirting. When you smile and banter with your male colleagues at work, or joke with the dude at the deli counter, you are engaging in innocent forms of flirting. This is not the type of flirting that can get a man to follow your scent the way a trained dog sniffs out scent. But it is a good place to start if you are an extremely shy woman.

Social Flirting

In contrast, social flirting is an indication of interest. It is like telling a man, "I see you, I think you see me too. I wonder where this will lead." You can do this by casting a sidelong gaze, accidentally brushing up against a guy you like, bumping into him several times in one night (accidentally, of course), or extending your goodbyes a little longer than usual. In subsequent chapters, we shall go into the details of how to flirt and we'll discuss more on this. But for now, understand that if you have an interest in a guy, social flirting is where you should start sending him the right signal and in the right quantity too. Too much sexual overtures and he may begin to think you are merely teasing him. On the other hand, too little sexual overtures and he will think of you as just a friend.

Private Flirting

This sets the stage for full-blown sexual innuendo because it is a type of flirting done one-on-one with a man who already gets your message loud and clear. This type of flirting can quickly lead to seduction. This is where the eye, lips, mouth, and other parts of the body including words are combined to send unmistakably powerful sexual signals to a man. Private flirting does not "wonder where things will lead," it knows exactly where things are headed.

Flirting: The Rules (Principles)

When I first began studying the art of flirting, I was eager to know what rules there were to follow. I wanted to understand what I needed to do and what I should avoid. I was itching to know the various techniques of flirting and seduction. But like any anxious young woman, I neglected something very important: the principles of flirting. When you hear the word "rule" you probably expect to read dos and don'ts. But what I term "flirting rules" are more like principles.

Techniques can change, they can be improved upon, and they can become obsolete, but universal principles don't change. Applying techniques without understanding the principles underlying those techniques can make you frustrated when you are not seeing the results you expected. That is a blind application at best. A proper understanding of the flirting principles will guide you on the most appropriate technique to apply when in any dating situation, and it can also help you to tweak or modify any technique to suit a particular situation. So, here are the fundamental principles of flirting. Indeed, they are simple and fun rules to remember.

Rule Number 1: Tune into Your Body

Flirting is not just something you do to someone; it is more about how you connect with yourself. When you understand this, you'll free yourself from the burden of doing things to impress men or other people in general, especially when it has to do with your sexuality. Instead, you'll do things to connect with your true self. Flirting is about embracing your feelings and letting them be expressed freely. The first rule of flirting is to tune into your sensuality and follow your pleasure. Allow yourself to be more attuned to your five senses so that you can become your bold, loving, and authentic self. In other words, when you interact with people (men in particular), become aware of any sexual feeling in your body no matter how small or faint the feeling is. Embracing this sexual feeling in totality without thinking of it as inappropriate will help you become comfortable to express that sexuality.

Activity: Here are things you can do to help you embrace your body and tune into your sensuality.

1. Light scented candles in your bathroom and let the aroma fill you up. Take daytime baths preferably bubble baths. Feel the warmth of the water on your skin and let the sound of the bubbles bursting on your skin hold your attention.

2. Treat yourself to a nice sensual massage. Become fully aware of the different sensations you feel as the masseurs or masseuse runs their fingers all over your beautiful body. Notice how each sensation feels and in what part of your body you feel it.

3. Listen to some classical music, preferably with your headphones on and your eyes closed. Allow your imagination to carry you to places you've never been before while you listen.

4. Buy silky nightwear and let your sense of touch relish the feel of its texture on your skin.

5. Gently touch and caress yourself. As you touch yourself, learn to listen to what your body craves. Have a little chat with your vagina. Ask her (your vagina) what she wants and listen for her response. It's okay if you don't get any intuitive response. The idea is to center yourself using this unique mindfulness meditation technique.

Note: Think of your sensuality as anything that causes you to experience physical pleasure. Whether it is a smell, colors, or the way your skin feels against a touch, permit yourself to fully embrace the sensations that life offers you. There's much pressure from society on us, women, to make us think and feel bad, shame or guilt for embracing and exploring our sensuality. Breaking free from such limiting thoughts is your first step to experiencing true freedom and becoming a woman who radiates loving and positive energy. You will also find that men, women and even children alike, are attracted to your magnetic presence because you exude something that they want to connect with.

Rationale for activity: Flirting is done to attract. You can't possibly want to attract someone to a body you are ashamed of. If anything, you would prefer not to be noticed because you are not comfortable in your own skin. The more comfortable you are in your feminine body, the more confident you are about your body and its sensations, the better you'll be at radiating that confidence to others. A woman who is attuned to her sensuality can send out magnetic signals in the form of eye contact, teasing someone, smiling, and even asking for help. But a woman who is ashamed of her sensuality tends to hide or send out the wrong signals.

Rule Number 2: Creative Visualization

If your mind is clouded with worries and fears of rejection or not being noticed, you will likely shoot yourself in the foot in your attempt at flirting. The second rule is to always visualize yourself with the man or men you want and open your heart to receive the attention. If you tell yourself that no man can possibly be interested in you, even when you find yourself in the perfect situation to flirt, your negative self-talk will prevent you from behaving flirtatiously. And even when you do, it is a half-hearted attempt.

Activity: To help you fill your mind with empowering thoughts about dating and relationships, do this exercise.

1. Sit in an upright position or lay flat on your back.

2. Breathe in deeply and exhale slowly.

3. Let your eyes close softly.

4. Picture a scenario with the man or men you'll like to attract.

5. Imagine that there is a flirtation dial right in front of your heart. Use your imagination to turn up the dial and attract the attention of those in your scenario.

6. Remain in this state of creative visualization for about five minutes and relish every conversation, sensation, and loving thought that crosses your mind.

7. Remember to approach this exercise with an attitude of fun and excitement rather than trying to make something happen. Think of it as your secret escape from reality because, indeed, what many of us women need is more fantasy, not more reality.

Note: It may seem silly at first to just sit and play with your imagination, especially if you are new to visualization. But its positive impact on your self-confidence is amazing. Don't dismiss this exercise no matter how silly it appears to you.

Rationale for activity: Success and failure all starts in your head. If you can see it in your mind's-eye, you can make it come true in your physical reality.

Rule Number 3: Reconnect with Your Sexuality

Sexuality is not something that you should only let out of its cage when you meet someone you like and want to date. Your sexuality is yours and is not dependent on any external circumstance or event. Own your sexuality. The third rule of flirting is to reconnect with your sexuality.

Activity: Engage in any of the following activities. You are welcome to think of other similar activities that can help you reconnect with your sexuality.

1. Put on your favorite music and simply dance to it. You don't have to be a good dancer, just let yourself loose and dance like no one is watching.

2. Do some grocery shopping and have a cooking fiesta.

3. Invite some friends over for dinner and wine. Make sure to get your friends to talk openly about your vaginas, sex and flirting, but downplay relationship drama. It's not a gathering for

mourning or lamenting over heartbreaks. Just have a good evening full of fun with your close friends.

Note: If you host an evening get-together with a few friends, don't be too surprised if your inbox gets bombarded the next day with praises, happy messages, and even questions from your friends. You may get texts or emails like, "What got into you?" "That's a side of you I've never seen… and I'm so loving it!" "Best get-together ever! Let's do this more often."

Rationale for activity: We are sexual beings but often want to shy away from our sexuality so that we can conform to society's standards. Reconnecting to your sexuality allows you to embrace the whole of your being just the way you are without censorship or judgment. Until you do, you'll keep looking for external approval from society to dictate to you how and when to be happy.

Let me quickly add that although these rules or principles are important to remember, flirting is not calculus. So remember to relax and have fun. There's no need to be all worked up because you want to flirt with your long-time crush or a total stranger. The goal is to create more fun in your life, not to put yourself under undue tension.

Flirting: The Benefits

Imagine what our world would look like without flirting. Heck, there'll be no world to begin with. Flirting is fundamental to the survival of the human species. We'll very quickly stop falling in love without flirting and that would be a huge threat to reproduction.

Flirting is not just about getting laid, although it could very well be about that. I mean, who doesn't want to have good sex and lots of fun? But besides sex and fun, there are other not-so-apparent benefits of flirting that can make you a better woman and even improve your overall outlook on life.

If having a good time with your dream man (whatever "good time" means for you) is the main dish of flirting, consider these benefits as the dessert or the icing on the flirting cake.

1. **Flirting helps you unwind:** Hanging out with friends after work exposes you to other men outside your work environment. You will feel much better about yourself and escape whatever stress or burden you've been carrying around all day.

2. **It can boost your self-esteem**: It feels so good when I know that men find me interesting, especially in a sexy way. I know a lot of women feel that way too. Flirting with men makes you feel wanted. That in itself makes you more confident in yourself because you must be doing something right to make someone interested in you. If you are a shy woman, I strongly encourage you to start with public flirting. When men become responsive, you'll notice a boost in your self-confidence, then you can up your game to social flirting and eventually private flirting.

3. **It makes you become a better person**: A woman who thinks no one is interested in her is likely to care less about her physical appearance; after all, nobody notices her. But if she is aware that someone is taking a special interest in her and that someone is a man, perhaps her long-time crush, she'll start to be more deliberate about her physical appearance and how she carries herself. She'll start to be picky about her dress, hair, and how she comports herself especially when there's an opposite-sex present. She becomes more self-aware and is likely to behave better because she is driven by a desire to be noticed in a positive light.

Generally, flirting will encourage you to put your best foot forward in anything you do.

4. **Flirting can encourage new and healthy habits**: If the man you desire is sexy, hot, and good-looking, you are very likely to start changing your attitude toward working out more and eating healthily more often. If you are withdrawn and shy but the man you want to flirt with is more extroverted, you may start considering going out more to give you the chance to catch his attention.

5. **It improves your communication even if you are already in a relationship**: It spices things up and rekindles the spark between you and your current partner. You are able to open up more to your partner and communicate in clearer terms. And if you are not yet in a relationship, flirting can help you communicate better verbally and nonverbally.

Let me bring this chapter to an end with a quote from Cate Mackenzie, a psychotherapist, love coach, artist, couples counselor, and psychosexual therapist. Mackenzie was quoted in a UK *Psychologies* blog as saying, "A woman who is a conscious and practiced flirt is learning the mastery of relationships and her environment. She knows how to use the force of love to be delightful and enticing. She creates a waterfall of deliciousness for herself and others" (Mackenzie, 2018).

Chapter 2

How Men Think

Humans have been socialized, but that doesn't take away our basic biological programming. This is why you'll notice that when a woman walks by a group of busy men, all activities seem to magically come to a temporal halt regardless of how important the activities are. Even if it is just one guy working his head off in his office, once a woman he considers attractive steps in, he'll momentarily pause and his ability to think rationally is frozen even if for a fraction of a second. His biological instinct (sexual impulse) temporarily takes over his mind and distracts his attention from whatever it was he was doing before. But this does not mean he is interested in the woman or that he will act on the impulse even if he is interested. The point is a man's biological programming is ever alive and continues to impact his behavior irrespective of social conditioning. A woman doesn't have to put in too much effort to get a man's attention—they are programmed to respond to us anyway. However, getting a man goes beyond just getting his attention.

To successfully flirt with any guy or even seduce him, you need to understand how he thinks. This does not mean spending extensive periods understudying him as though you were studying for a Ph.D. It, however, means having the basic knowledge about how men generally tend to think. But first, let me make two things clear. First, this book is about how to flirt, not about how men think. I am only bringing men's way of thinking into the picture because I am assuming that you are a heterosexual woman who wants to flirt with a man. Secondly, men are pretty simple and straightforward. There's usually nothing too complex about the average man. However, many of the things in this chapter are generalizations about men. So, don't assume that they are absolutely correct for every man.

The Male Psyche

The phrase *"cut to the chase"* is, in my opinion, a masculine phrase. Men generally don't have the patience for details, especially regarding relationships. This is one of the reasons a man can't understand why a woman would spend hours in front of a mirror. When a typical husband asks his wife what a repairman said, for example, what he is asking for is the bottom line, the cost of the repairs. But a typical wife would go into every detail of what the repairman said. That usually bores the man silly. Men generally like to get things over and done with as soon as possible. It's like something inside of them keeps asking "What's next?"

This reminds me of the 2001 movie A Beautiful Mind, where John Nash (played by Russell Crowe) "arrogantly" said to a lady who was obviously flirting with him, "I don't exactly know what I am required to say in order for you to have intercourse with me. But could we assume that I said all that? I mean essentially we are talking about fluid exchange right? So could we go just straight to the sex?" That earned him a well-deserved smack on his face.

I am not saying that men are usually like Nash, but that's a clear example (even if it's exaggerated) of how simple (logical?) men's psyche's are. No intricacies, sophistication, or shades of gray—just black or white.

Men's brains come equipped with only the basic requirements so they usually are not open to remembering every detail of every event that happens. Inside a man's brain are compartments for the different aspects of his life. When he discusses an issue, he goes to the compartment meant for that particular issue and focuses only on that issue. There is a particular compartment in his brain that is empty. This is where he spends his quiet time when he is stressed. When you see a man engaged in a seemingly brain-dead activity for hours, is most likely in his special empty compartment.

On the other hand, women have lots of extra memory attached to their brains, so they usually remember lots of details. Inside a woman's brain, there are no compartments, instead, every aspect of her life is connected to every other aspect and is usually powered by her emotions. She can switch from one topic to another randomly and seamlessly, which is why we tend to multitask more than men.

While men tend to be more rational, analytical, and logical, women lean more toward emotional reasoning—we generally "feel" and are heart-centered while men generally "think" and are head-centered. Men often prefer to be left alone when stressed. They drift into the special compartment containing nothing and remain there to get over their stress. Women, on the other hand, tend to want to talk about what bothers them. Trying to make a man talk when he prefers to be left alone can lead to conflict in a relationship.

But what does all of this have to do with flirting? Here's the link. It doesn't matter how many hours and effort a lady spends trying to look expensive, hot and attractive, a man does not have too much time to analyze all the details. You are either attractive or not; there's no in between. When a man sees a woman, his logical brain is quick to classify her into one of the many compartments in his brain: classy, tease, cheap, hot, for keeps, a turnoff, and so on. If you don't fall into his definition of "attractive," you can put in all the efforts to get his attention, but that won't make him desire you even if he notices you. This is particularly frustrating for a woman if she becomes obsessive about trying to get the attention of the man she wants. To make a man interested in you, you must first discover what his compartment for an attractive, interesting, and desirable woman looks like.

If you are able to answer these questions, it will go a long way to help you figure out what your ideal man's compartment for a desirable woman looks like.

- Where does he hang out? Who does he hang out with?
- Is he the outgoing social type, or the introverted avoid-the-crowd type of guy?
- Is he into physical fitness, or he doesn't mind his protruding belly?
- What does his social media profile say about him?

Knowing these things will help you put in effort in the right direction and save you the headache of shouting into the wind. In the next chapter, I shall go into more detail about this. However, if you are not interested in establishing a strong connection with a man, you don't need to put in too much effort figuring out anything about his psyche. Work on making him respond to his biological programming and you are likely to have lots of fun together even if it's just for one night.

What Attracts a Man

Every man has his own truth, but there are certain attitudes in women that men find attractive. Do your best to develop a few of these attitudes if you don't already have them to help you improve your chances of being attractive to not just men, but everyone you interact with.

1. **Smile**: One of the first nonverbal cues that show a man your interest in him is a warm smile. It indicates openness and can make a man easily start a conversation with you. To build a killer smile, practice different smiles using one of the greatest manmade tools every woman has—the mirror. Stand in front of your mirror and give yourself a sly smile, a smirk, a broad smile, and so on. Note the one that makes you look more welcoming, open, and genuine and use it for the man you truly want to be with. Reserve the rest for other situations such as telling a man off, coming off as mysterious, or when you're trying to hide your interest in a man. Although you can use any type of smile you choose for any situation, what is important is knowing when to use a genuine smile. A genuine smile touches the eyes. Putting on a fake smile makes you look desperate and can quickly turn a man off.

2. **A Positive Attitude and Open Body Language**: People with positive attitudes generally have open body language. Notice the person who has people paying attention to him or her in the room, and you'll see that they most likely have open body language. They don't have their arms crossed against their chests or keep a bland

expression. Practice wearing smiles that touch your eyes—that's how to have bright eyes. When you interact with people, practice open arm gestures instead of keeping your hands in your pants pocket. A positive attitude is contagious and acts like a magnet that attracts people (both men and women) to you. We'll take a more detailed look into body language in a subsequent chapter.

3. **Exude High Energy and Confidence**: Many women often mistake arrogance for confidence. To be clear, arrogance is being brash and brazen; confidence, on the other hand, is being firm and assertive. While there is some level of confidence hidden under such behavior, arrogance usually shows up as being rude. Men generally love a confident woman but will most definitely stay away from a cocky woman. Being confident doesn't mean you are perfect. It is an acknowledgment of your imperfections as well as your beauty, smartness, sexiness, and, of course, your humorous side. When you are all over a man, the message he gets is that you lack confidence in yourself and you are desperate. Even if you are head over heels for a man, act as if you don't need him. It's difficult sometimes, I know. But you have to activate the hunter instinct in him so that he can

chase after you. Offering yourself to him on a platter of gold when you are not yet into a relationship will make him highlight, drag, and drop you in his brain's compartment labeled "cheap." When you walk into a room, let your steps exude confidence—hold your shoulders back walk as if you own the entire room.

4. **Kindness**: Small and random acts of kindness are often noticed by men. Again, the biological programming of a man makes him more open to a woman who tends to behave motherly to others. Kindness is one of such motherly traits. When you are with the man you like and want to attract, find opportunities to display kindness. Treat the waiter or waitress with respect, offer a hand to the elderly, wave at children, do him little favors, and so on. In a world where being rude or less concerned about others is almost the norm, showing respect and kindness to him and others would make him itch to know you better.

5. **A Sense of Humor**: When you laugh genuinely, you unconsciously tell a man that you feel free in his presence and that you enjoy his company. Tell jokes, laugh when he tells jokes, let yourself loose and laugh at your mistakes. When you respond to humor, you peel back all the sophistication of

being a lady and give a man a glimpse into the real you. Which man wouldn't be curious to see more of the "behind-the-curtain" version of you?

Different Strokes for Different Folks

Although I have described men in general terms, all men are not the same (as we women often want to believe). In some cases, you'll find men who are completely opposite to how I have described them in this chapter, which goes to prove that all men are not the same. The point here is to find out exactly what applies to the particular man you are interested in. Of course, if you are not interested in building a long-term relationship with a man, you can go ahead and attract his attention alone. It is quite easy to do that; lick your lips, look helpless, flick your hair, and so on. I'll get into the nitty-gritty of all much that later. Doing any of those can get his attention, and you might even have great sex together or whatever idea of fun you want. But if what you truly desire is to get a man helplessly in love with you, focus on knowing what works for him particularly. Then you can begin to entice him along those lines. If you generalize things, you may not be so lucky and you'll find that you are trying to bait a fish with dog treats because you assumed it was a dog.

Chapter 3

Holding His Attention Long Enough

Let's flip the script for a minute. Imagine a guy you've never seen before walking up to you and pulling down his pants. Your reaction will most likely be that of shock rather than being turned on (unless you're in a freaky mood). Now, how do you think a man would react to you if you did the same? Because men generally are more attracted sex doesn't mean he will be turned on by a total stranger shoving her boobs in his face or taking off her pants in front of him. Instead of activating his sexual instinct, that behavior is likely to activate his protective instinct. He'll try to cover you and get you help (assuming he's a civilized man) instead of being turned on. Of course, the environment and mood can change how things play out. In a wild party or carnival, anything goes. But I'm not referring to parties and funfairs. I'm talking about everyday situations.

Getting a man's attention is one thing, getting him attracted to you is another ball game entirely. I've seen lots of women who feel that they are invisible to the man of their dreams do unusual things (sometimes, crazy things) to get his attention. The problem with attention is it usually is short-lived and does not automatically mean he is attracted to you. So, if you think what you'll get in this book is merely a bunch of superficial pieces of advice such as flick your hair, dress sexily and so on, well, that's not going to happen. Men can easily see through such acts and can quickly conclude that you are desperate and insecure. This would leave you more frustrated, bitter, and even make you start to doubt yourself. Even if you do get a man's attention with such moves, it will not necessarily make him fall head over heels for you.

If what you are looking for is a long-term loving relationship, the process is to get a man's attention, make him attracted to you, and then flirt with him. Heck, seduce him like crazy but only after he becomes attracted to you. On the other hand, if what you're looking for is to have a fling then skip the attraction part. Start by flirting with him and then get laid.

In other words, first, get him attracted, and then flirt with him if you want a long-term relationship. Or begin by flirting with him to get his attention if all you want is a fling.

To Get His Attention Avoid These Mistakes

It is important that you know the common mistakes that most of us women make when trying to get a guy's attention. Avoiding these mistakes can improve your chances of attracting genuine interest from a man instead of getting only fleeting attention.

1. **Not knowing your next move after getting his attention**: So, you've made all the right moves and he has noticed you. Now what? What do you say to him when he's standing or sitting next to you? What's your next move? Smile sheepishly and wait indefinitely for him to say something? What if he does start a conversation, where do you want to go with the conversation? If you are going to get him hooked, you need to figure out within the first few minutes of your interaction if he's single, if he's there with someone else, if he's straight, and if he is really interested in you. Once you have his attention and

you are sure he's the type of guy you want to date, make it abundantly clear that you are interested in him by being flirty.

2. **Trying to make a man jealous**: It is immature to intentionally make a man jealous just to get his attention. Flirting with his friend to make him jealous is not a classy thing to do, and neither is having your friends tell his friends that you find him attractive. Younger women make this mistake a lot of the time, but women of every age are also found wanting in this aspect. Quit acting like a naïve teenage girl. Subsequently, I'll show you more matured ways to use his friends when you are trying to get his attention and it does not involve manipulation.

3. **Assuming that a few dates automatically mean a serious relationship**: If you've gone on a few dates with a guy, it doesn't indicate a declared relationship or a commitment for life. Understand that dating is a process that is intended to make you both see if there's something that clicks for you. Avoid getting carried away too soon because he agreed to a few dates. You may have gotten his attention quite all right, but still, it doesn't mean he is into you. Ladies tend to allow their emotions decide for them when it comes to

dates and relationships. Be that woman who is strong enough to put that part of her in check when she is meeting a guy she finds attractive.

4. **Assuming that attention equals attraction**: Just about anything a woman does can get a man's attention, but that doesn't mean he is attracted to the woman. The way you smile, laugh, carry yourself, heck, even the way you tilt your head when you listen to someone talk can get a man's attention. But would that be enough to make him want to date you or go into a relationship with you? And even if he's been on a date with you because you held his attention long enough to make him want to have dinner with you, it still isn't a confirmation that he is attracted to you. A man can spend the evening with you, yet his reaction to you is cold and distant. If he is struggling to keep his attention on you and other people or his phone while he is with you, quit wasting your time on the wrong man—he's not attracted to you.

Calling His Attention

Before a man becomes attracted to you, you'll need to get his attention first. So, here are some classy ways to get a man's attention. These techniques work the same way a dog whistle does—it makes no sound to the human ear, but the dog hears it loud and clear.

1. **Give attention to his friend**: Earlier, I mentioned that there are better ways to get a guy's attention using his friends without making him feel jealous. It is by initially paying attention to his friends instead of him. But if you use this strategy, remember to not overdo it because your primary target is him and not his friend or friends.

   If a guy you want is with a friend, the friend is likely to feel like an annoying appendage if you go directly to the man you want and start a conversation. So, focus first on the friend. You will be putting the friend at ease because he'll not feel you want to get him out of the way to chat up his attractive buddy. It also gives room for group interaction. And including everyone in the interaction can also make his friend encourage him to go for you if you are a likable person.

2. **Friend or follow him on social media**: When a man sees a friend requests from a lady on his

social media page such as Facebook, for example, his mind is likely to go, "Hmm... that's interesting." He may accept a fellow man's friends request without going through their profile, but will likely check out a lady's profile and even zoom in on her pictures while at it. It is biology, and it is encoded in his genetic makeup. You are likely to call his attention to yourself by the simple act of adding him up on Twitter, Instagram, Facebook, Snapchat, or whatever social media you both use.

Let me quickly add that this can be a very wrong move if you don't do it right. Not too many guys are into social media as ladies are, and trying to snoop around his social media page may turn you into an overly eager lady who wants to pounce on him. Resist the urge to leave him eager messages on social media even if you find him very attractive. That way, you'll play it cool and give him the impression that you befriend just about anyone you meet on social media. You will reduce your risk of getting rejected or seen as a stalker if you put a leash on how you interact with him on social media.

3. **Note what he posts on social media**: You can use his interest on social media to draw his attention to you. I did not say chat him on social

media about his interests; he will know you just read something on his social media page and you are desperate about talking to him. Simply note what he says on social media and use that as a conversation starter the next time you are with him or simply make a positive comment about his interest the next time he's with you. To make it more attractive, say it casually like something you'll say in passing. If you make it a major point of discussion, he'll see through the act. For example, if he posts something on social media about basketball, maybe about his team winning a championship, it makes you know he likes basketball and you know his team. The next time you meet him, you can casually mention how great that team was in their last game. That could be a strong rapport builder.

But for this to work well, you have to make sure that you bring up only things that you genuinely like about his social media posts or at least things you don't hate. If you don't like basketball, for example, and he's a big fan of basketball, look for something else about his interest that you like or do not feel negative about. Faking interest in something you don't like is an uphill task you'll not be able to keep up with.

4. **Display your natural abilities**: It is difficult to keep up with pretense, but a lot easier to be natural. Embracing and being yourself is, perhaps, one of the sexiest things you can do to get a man's attention. There is no unnatural effort—you're just being you. For example, if you meet a guy you like at a music club and you are good with any instrument, you could play your heart out while making sure he is paying attention. If you are a gifted dancer, you can dance alone or with a partner while he is paying attention. Seize that opportunity to include some sexy moves in your dance steps. If you are good at public speaking and you met a guy you like at a company event, for example, you could volunteer to give a dazzling presentation (don't overdo it, though). He will notice you and is likely to want to get to know you more.

Getting Him Hooked

Getting a man's attention is only the chase; the kill is in getting him strongly attracted to you. And to do that, you need to go beyond superficial acts and really connect with what makes your ideal man tick. That is the surest way to get a man truly attracted to you.

Target His Lovemap

We all have what psychologists call the lovemap. The lovemap is a subconscious guide about our perfect partner. It is built little by little over the course of our life. A large part of our lovemap is built around our unmet needs, especially emotional needs. If a guy grows up with parents who are always fighting because one of them is an alcoholic, he is not likely to be impressed with a partner who drinks a lot. His dream woman would be someone more sober and loving. A guy who was bullied a lot as a kid would probably grow to desire a woman that reassures, admires, and compliments him for being both mentally and physically strong.

When you discover a man's lovemap, you can make him strongly attracted to you because you are speaking a language that his subconscious understands. You are fulfilling a secret desire he has that he may not even be aware of because it is a subliminal desire. A man's subconscious recognizes behaviors in a woman that can compensate for the things he lacks. Meeting a man's unmet emotional needs has a greater impact on him than merely flicking your hair and licking your lips. If you get him hooked through his lovemap, it becomes easier for licking of lips and other flirting moves to make him go weak in the knees. If you don't meet a guy's lovemap specification, flirting with him is not likely to make him attracted to you.

I'll suggest the following ways to target his lovemap:

1. Find out what his unmet needs are. You'll get some clue from his social media page, his hobbies, what attracted him to his hobbies, major life challenges and setbacks, the type of relationship he has with his family and friends, and his upbringing.

2. Ask him carefully worded questions aimed at eliciting information that can help you know his lovemap specifications. You could carefully chip in questions during conversations such as what childhood memories he cherishes most? What the happiest time of his life was? What are the strangest things he's done in his life? In order not to spook him, make your questions appear playful. You could mask pretty deep questions by playing saying things like, "Let's assume that I could magically make anything go away from your life. Perhaps it's someone you find annoying, something in your past you'll like to erase, or something happening in society you'll like to change—anything at all. What would that be?" Being playful about the questioning process will

make him feel at ease in answering them. If you make it sound like an interview, he may not be willing to divulge such information to you. Moreover, playfulness opens his imagination to explore things in his life he would like to change.

3. When you discover his lovemap specifications, begin to gradually work on meeting those needs. For example, if you find that he is into bodybuilding because he was bullied as a child, you could say things that make him feel strong physically and emotionally. Tell him how great and strong his physique is. He will gradually begin to feel strongly drawn to you emotionally without even knowing why. You are essentially compensating for something he feels he is lacking—physical and emotional strength. Don't be surprised when he starts telling you things like, "You make me feel complete."

4. Now flirt with him. If you get a man's attention and eventually build strong attraction, don't let it go to waste. Give him some encouragement. Show him that you are as attracted to him as he is to you. Stirring his biological programming along with his lovemap is like adding fuel to an already ignited fire—it will burn hotter.

Is This Ethical?

Some people would think it is manipulative to make a man fall in love with you. But if you genuinely care about a man and intend to treat them right, support their dream just as you know they will also support yours, and even possibly build a life together, then nudging them into falling in love with you is ethical in my opinion. Women who are already in a relationship can also use their man's lovemap to strengthen their relationship.

However, if your intention is just to prove a point, to stroke your ego, or simply to get into bed with them, then you are taking undue advantage of their lovemap and that is unethical. If you are not interested in sharing a loving relationship with a man, stick with flirting and seduction instead of making him fall in love with you. You can have all the fun you want with as many men as you wish without necessarily going to the trouble of making them fall helplessly in love with you. You wouldn't want a man to take advantage of you in that way now, would you?

Bottom Line

Getting a man's attention and making him take a genuine interest in you requires some effort, but it is a worthwhile effort. The attraction may not happen instantly but if you keep working on it, it will eventually pay off. You don't need to do every tip you read in this chapter or book before you get the man of your choice. I will suggest that you stick with the tips that resonate with you and leave out the rest. It is also important to not lose yourself in the process of attracting a man. Stay true to your values and what is most important to you. And most of all, be confident in your ability to attract just the right man for yourself. Your self-confidence grows as you get to practice these tips to get a guy's attention. It doesn't matter if the attention morphs into an attraction or not. What is important at the beginning is to be able to get men's attention at will. Before long, you become so good at it that men will become attracted to you even when you are not trying to get them. This happens because as you keep feeling good and confident about your ability, you'll continue to refine your style and efforts. Flirting will become easier for you, seduction will follow naturally, and the right things to say will become second nature. In short, men will find you irresistible.

Chapter 4

What if He's not Showing Interest?

Okay, so you've followed the script and done everything right, yet the man you're dying to attract isn't reciprocating what you feel for him. Or you've had him for a while and he's beginning to lose interest in you. Or you're simply not sure if he's into you or not. What should you do next? Before I show you exactly what you can do if the man you want is not interested in you, let's quickly see some of the signs that'll make you know for sure he's just not into you.

Surefire Signs That Says a Man is not Interested in You

First of all, if you had to Google "How to know if a guy is interested in you or not" then it's most likely that your man is fast losing interest in you or he isn't into you to begin with. You deserve a man who doesn't leave you wondering where things stand between you both.

If a guy is showing any of these signs, it means he's not interested in you:

1. **Your personal life, goals, and viewpoints mean little to him**: A man who is interested in you would want to know you better. He'll go beyond the usual "How are you?" surface question. He'll want to know your life's goals, things you like and don't like, your viewpoints, and even your family. If he's not showing such a level of interest in you, he is not that into you.

2. **He's not making any sexual advances**: Do you remember the biological programming we talked about in the previous chapter? Well, if you're dating a guy who doesn't expressively tells you that he's staying off sex until marriage or that he intends to remain celibate, his biological programming will make him want to at least hug you a bit longer than necessary (that is, if he's got a lot of self-control). No matter how respectful or nice a man is, if he is physically attracted to you, he will want to have sex with you, kiss you, touch you in the most affectionate ways or hold your

hand lovingly. But if he's not making any of these moves, he considers you as a friend and nothing more.

3. **He's distracted when he's with you**: If he's always chatting with other people while he's with you, or he is always playing a game on his phone when you around, or he prefers giving other people attention instead of you, you're a bore to him.

4. **You're not included in his future**: When a guy finds you interesting, you'll hear things like, "Let's have dinner at my favorite restaurant next weekend," or "How would you like to come with me to the Yankees game next month? I got two tickets." If he is not including you in any of his future plans, he is probably not envisioning you and him together in any foreseeable future and that's not a good sign.

5. **He treats you just like any other woman**: If a man is not treating you as special or is treating you with less regard than he does to other women, he is not interested in you. His words and actions should make you feel special, desired, appreciated, and wanted. If all that is missing or you notice he's using the same words and actions for other women

too, it's probably his usual way of talking to all ladies—you included. There's nothing special about it. When a man is attracted to you or is interested in you, there's just no hiding it. He may not do special things for and with you every day, but for most of your time together, you'll feel special. Men generally don't hide it when they are interested. I mean, just look at a guy who is sexually attracted to a lady and you'll see his sexual member physically attesting to the fact. A woman knows she digs a guy but will cover it up because that's just what we do. Not so with a man; he'll chase after you because that's what men do also. If he's not making you feel special to him, if he's not doing things that make you feel different from the other women in his life (his sisters, mother, and female friends), there's no second-guessing the fact that he's just not interested in you.

6. **He stays out of touch**: In this time and age, there are innumerable ways an interested guy can stay in touch with you. If he's not calling, emailing, texting, Facebooking, Skyping, tweeting, or using any of the several communication channels to stay in touch with you for considerably long periods, he's definitely not thinking about you. If you reach

out to him and he doesn't respond because he's busy or for some other reason, he'll get back to you on time and he'll certainly apologize or offer some explanation. Generally, a guy who is interested in your will respect you enough to keep the lines of communication open because he thinks you are very important to him. If he doesn't, you are not that important to him.

7. **He doesn't seem to remember important things about you**: As I've mentioned in the previous chapter, men generally don't have time to remember details, but a man that is head over heels for you will acquire additional memory space in his brain and label that compartment "my special one." When a man is interested in you, he will remember you because you are his topmost priority. He'll remember your birthday, and if you've been together for a while, he'll remember your anniversary. He'll want to spend holidays with you or at least call you during the holidays. The significant events of his life and your life will be a shared celebration for him. If he's constantly forgetting or deliberating not treating things about you seriously, he simply is not interested in you beyond the surface level.

8. **He's always talking about his ex**: This is a clear indication that he's not yet over his ex. Staying with a man who is still hung up on his ex is settling for second place. You are worth more than that. Let him go.

Reasons Why He's on the Fence

There are quite some reasons a man may not be interested in you, despite you doing all the right things. But let us consider the top three reasons.

1. **He is just a manipulator**: A manipulator knows exactly what he wants, and it's certainly not you. He wants is to have sex with you while still doing the same thing with as many naïve women he can manipulate. But what's manipulative about it is that he continues to trick you with "I need more time to figure it out," when, in fact, he has it figured out right from the beginning. A manipulator is a booty guy. He doesn't call or text you during the day to know how your day is going. You'll only get his text or calls late at night because he's not interested in a relationship.

   No matter how attractive you find a manipulator or a booty guy, dump him and move on. If he is acting this way from the onset, imagine what you'll have to deal with if your relationship becomes official. You need to end that relationship before it starts. Stop flirting with him or even trying to seduce him. Turn off your charm and become assertive in kicking him out of your life for good. This is the only way you can open your heart to other men who will not play games with your heart.

2. **He is genuinely confused**: A guy may really like you, but he's distracted by other factors in his life. It could be that he's about to relocate before meeting the most amazing woman (you) he's ever known, and he's at a crossroad—to stay with you or to move. It even more complicated and confusing for him if the move is due to his job or career. He finds himself between the devil and the deep blue sea. Even if it's for study purposes, he may not want to start a distant relationship. It could also be that he finds you attractive and he likes you, but his ex is still trying to get him back. Here's how you'll know if a guy is genuinely confused about getting into a relationship with you. You feel an actual strong emotional connection to him when he's with you. Both of you feel the bond, and he's generally honest with you. But when he's not around you, you feel a sense of

detachment as if he's deliberately pulling away from you. He'll always be undecided or unnecessarily tentative about plans with you. You will feel the barrier between you even though you can sense that he wants you.

The best way to get through this is to talk to him about what you've observed. Talk about it openly and honestly and see if you both can work out something. If his reasons don't look good, there will be no need to put more energy into the relationship.

3. **He wants to know you better**: Not everyone has the same timing for decision-making when it comes to relationships. You see a guy and you find him attractive, and then you make moves to make him notice you because you already like the much you've noticed about him. Keep in mind that he may not be a quick judge of character or he's suffered some terrible heartbreak in the past. One quick way to know if he's on the fence because he wants to know you better is if you haven't known each other for very long.

Give him time. But be aware that you cannot wait on a man indefinitely. Let him understand your definition of "enough time." If he can't make up his mind about you both being an item after your "enough time," he probably doesn't trust you enough to be in a relationship with.

What to Do if He is Not Interested in You

Do you remember how I said men tend to be more logical while we tend to be more emotional? Well, being emotional about rejection can drive you into self-pity, anger, and other self-destructive behaviors. To intelligently handle a man who is not interested in you, you'll have to play down the emotional reasoning and apply more logic using the following suggestions.

Respect His Decision and Respect Yours Too

When a man says "I'm not sure I'm ready for a relationship," that could be the worst thing any woman would ever want to hear. But instead of reacting angrily or telling him to go to hell, take a pause and breathe in and out a couple of times to center yourself. He may not be ready for a relationship or he specifically doesn't want a relationship with you. Whatever the case, you need to give him a response that shows that you truly care about him, but you also love yourself. Switching from a kind, loving, and affectionate lady to a venomous woman the very next minute will only confirm why he shouldn't enter into a relationship with you to begin with.

You could say something along this line: "I hear you and it's clear to me that you need to be by yourself for a while to figure out what's really important to you. Your happiness is important to me, and I do wish you will find what makes you truly happy even if that means being without me. I hope that I'll still be here when you are ready for a relationship, but until you figure out what you truly want, I can't be with someone who's not ready to be 100% with me."

Saying this will have a big impact on him in the following ways:

1. He's not sure if he wants to be in a relationship. But here you are being very sure about what you want (which doesn't include a confused guy). You're telling him that you're not going to "sell him anything." It's absolutely his choice to make.

2. You're making it okay for him to not want to be in a relationship with you. This takes away his power to push against whatever resistance it was he was expecting you to put up. Suddenly, he'll realize that his "unsure state" is not as attractive as he thought it was.

3. He'll see how pure and loving you are when you say you care about his happiness even if it means being without you. He knows he's about losing someone very dear and scarce to come by.

4. Telling him that you hope you'll still be around when he makes up his mind plants a seed of doubt in him. He knows he may not find everything he thinks he'll get with some other person. And when he comes back, you may be happily gone for good.

5. And, finally, you tell him how valuable you think and know you are when you say you want and deserve to be with someone who is 100% into you. You are telling him that you love and respect him, but you also love and respect yourself.

Responding this way tells him that even though you're not eager to lose him, it's his loss if he chooses to let you slip through his fingers.

Give Him Space

Showing a guy that you're crazy about him by leaving him a ton of messages, voicemails, and emails are choking. If he's not interested in you, the more you try—the more effort you put into getting him interested, the farther away you push him and the lesser your value gets before him. It may be tough, but resist the urge to keep texting him. And to make it easier for you, once he has made it abundantly clear that he is not interested in you, delete his contact, and unfriend and unfollow him if you are friends on social media. Remove anything that would tempt you to get in touch with him or look him up. It doesn't mean you should hate him; that would do you no good either. Use your energy and emotion for better things than hating on him.

Be Yourself

It is dangerous and always leads to more frustration to try to change yourself to suit a man. Be yourself, just as you'll want him to be himself. Trying to be someone else is very tiring—you don't want to embark on a journey that will get you nowhere. If a man likes you, you don't need to change yourself to enjoy the relationship. If your trusted friends and family start telling you that you are being someone else just to get a guy, take a pause and seriously consider your behaviors. Are you always making excuses for his behavior? Are you always reassuring yourself that he'll eventually come around? Being in a one-sided relationship to please a man just to keep him is slavery.

Manage Your Expectations

It is easy to get trapped in the hope that one day he'll realize his mistakes and come running back to you. Give that up. The only person who type of thinking hurts is you. You are only going to keep getting your hopes up and smashing them into pieces. Instead of looking forward to his text or calls where he'll say how wrong he was and how right you are, channel your energy to things that get in back in control of your emotions. Start each day with a positive outlook. Let your happiness come from how you behave, not on whether or not he reaches out to you. Let go of expecting him to come around. Release yourself from the pain of hope against all hope.

Quit Fighting Over Him

"If I can't have him, no one will!" Really? You are seriously considering a brawl to keep someone to yourself? You're worth more than that. If after doing everything possible, a man still thinks you're not worth his time, it's his loss. It can be a heartbreaking experience and you're welcome to grieve about it. But whatever you do, don't embarrass yourself by begging to be loved. Nothing makes a man think less of a woman than when she becomes needy, clingy, and displays very poor self-esteem. When a man wants to attract a woman, he's the needy one. But when a woman wants to attract a man, she makes herself the needed one. Don't ever forget that.

Realize You Can't Change Him

If you've been with a guy for a while and he's clearly not into you, let him be. Don't attempt to change him because you can't. It doesn't matter how much time, effort, money, love, and so on you've invested in him and the relationship, let it go. Don't fall into the trap of the Sunk Cost Fallacy—thinking that you've put in too much to let go. That will only leave more drained physically and emotionally. Realize that a man is who he is regardless of what you do. If he is not giving you what you want and you begin to have a feeling of changing him, recognize immediately that he is not what you want. Keep your focus on *what* you want in a man rather than on *who* you want a man to be. What you want is a man who will treat you as his top priority, respect, cherish, adore, and desire you. You want a man who thinks you are special and wants to be with you so badly. If a man is not doing these things that you want, no matter how hot he looks or how great you think he can be, he is not really what you want. Quit trying to make him into something he is clearly not. He may have the potential for all of and can even become that type of person for some other woman who he finds interesting but certainly not you. Let him go. It is not your flaw or imperfection that is making him act that way. It's just who he is. Instead of wasting your energy in pushing him to become someone he is not, concentrate on what you really want. Define what truly matters to you and stick with it.

Chapter 5

The Body Language of Flirting

This chapter is designed to show you how to activate what is already in you. As you read, allow yourself to visualize scenarios where you are applying these techniques. But avoid trying to memorize any move. Get out and stay out of your head when you want to flirt. Flow with your feelings and your body will automatically send the right signals. Stay in your head and your movements will be mechanical. A smile that touches the eyes comes from the heart, not the head. The same applies to other body language and nonverbal cues. You should read them to expose your mind to their usage but to use them effortlessly, you should allow the way you feel at any moment guide you on what move to make.

The Eyes

The eyes have been called the window to the soul. With it, you can see through anyone. Flirting without using the eyes is like sending signals randomly without a specific target. When you make eye contact, your signal has a direction and is aimed at a target.

How to Flirt with Your Eyes

To begin with, you need eyes to see who you want to flirt with. If what you see is pleasant to you and you want to call attention to yourself, start with making eye contact. Men generally miss the first flirting sign a woman gives. So you need to look at a man two or three times before he gets the message. But it goes beyond just looking or making eye contact. If you are in a crowded place, there's a high chance that your eyes will meet with a lot of people more than once. That is not flirting. To make it flirtatious, look at him until his gaze catches. Wait for one or two seconds before looking away. Stealing a look at a man you are interested in may make him feel he is being spied on instead of turning him on. Make sure your eyes meet for a few seconds before looking away. He will want to be sure, so wait for a few more minutes before making another eye contact, but this time accompany it with a smile. If you are flirting with someone you've never met before, avoid giving them a wink. That could portray you as being cheap or tactless. Reserve the wink for a man you have met a couple of times and with whom you would want to be more than just friends.

Using your eyes this way goes to the heart of flirting. Flirting is an attraction routine that thrives on the promise-withdraw method of arousing interest. With your eyes, you give someone your attention (the promise of interest), and then you look away (withdraw the promise), but then repeat the promise-withdraw dance again. This creates the sensation of tension-release- tension in the mind of your target. If he wasn't sure of your first eye contact, the second time coupled with a warm smile could only mean one thing: interest.

Practice Looking at People

Your eyes are usually the first avenues other people read or feel your energy. Whether you are out to flirt or not, when you walk into a room full of people remember to practice holding the gaze of those who turn to look at you. And smile too. Looking at someone without smiling can be misread as a sign of hostility because you are staring. The more times you practice deliberately holding people's gaze with a smile, the better you get at expressing yourself through your eyes. This is particularly helpful if you tend to be shy and avoid eye contact when interacting with people. Continue practicing, first, with people you are familiar with, and then gradually with total strangers. And soon, you will be able to call any man's attention simply by looking at him.

Head Movements

Nodding

Nodding may not seem like a flirting signal, but it conveys interest when used correctly. You can squint your eyes slightly while you nod a few times when he is talking with you. Nodding is particularly useful if you are trying to get a man's attention in a formal situation such as a business meeting. But you never can say where you'll find a good looking man who will take your breath away. You may not directly flirt with him at that moment, but your body language should convey your interest. Nodding and occasional smiles are some of such "innocent" signals that could give room to more meetings in a less formal situation where you can be more up-front with other sexually persuasive flirting signals.

Flip Your Hair

Consciously or unconsciously running your hand through your hair, twirling it, or flipping your hair over your shoulder are all signs of flirting that never gets old. Make sure your hair is neat and smells nice. The fragrance that lingers after you flip your hair will make him more attracted to you especially if he is sitting close to you.

Facial Expressions

The "Come-Hither" Look

Usually, when we experience intense pleasure, we tend to slightly raise our eyebrows at the same time lower our eyelids. This is known as the come-hither look. This facial expression is not exclusively reserved for the bedroom. When you give a man this look, it is a clear signal that you want him.

You can perfect your come-hither look by adding a sly smile (not a smile that shows your teeth). Stand in front of a mirror and practice several times to get the killer look you want.

Smile

Smiling is a gesture that invites or attracts people to you. A bland expression is not likely to get any man interested in you. Smiling makes you approachable. And it lights up your entire face especially if it is a genuine smile that reaches your eyes. Flash your man smiles to set him at ease and encourage him to go on with the chase. Look into his eyes when you smile to make your smile more effective. When you smile, remember to return your expression to normal. Pasting a smile on your face long after the reason for the smile is over will give you a ridiculous look.

Wink

A wink is rather an audacious move. Use it only when you are familiar with the man. Avoid using it more than once. Repeating winks makes you look creepy.

Mouthing a Kiss

Blow him a kiss if you are more daring. He will come looking for you even if you disappear after mouthing the kiss. I suggest that you use this sparingly. Wait until you are sure that he is really attracted to you and you really like him before blowing him a kiss. Ideally, you should first use other flirting signals and gauge his level of interest before mouthing him a kiss.

Pouting Your Lips

Pouting your lips as a sign of flirting is not the same as pursing in front of a camera. Here's a tip to give your lips the perfect pout. Try saying the word "blue" (silently of course). Adding colorful lipstick and slightly squint your eyes to enhance your pout. First, practice in front of a mirror until you get it right. You don't want to look like a fish when you pout. And you certainly don't want your man to think you are angry or sad.

Licking and Biting Your Lips

Licking your lips can convey interest. To make it more natural, make eye contact and then sip your drink. This is a perfect time to lick your lips without appearing unnatural. When you bit your lower lips without first making eye contact, a man might think you are uncomfortable or stressed. So, make sure to first engage his eyes before you slightly bite your lower lips. That way, he will get your message loud and clear.

Touching Him

Breaking the Touch Barrier

Initiating tactile touch is one of the clearest signals to a man indicating that you want to go beyond just a friendly conversation or professional relationship. But breaking the touch barrier is something a lot of women find difficult to do even when they are dying to touch him a man they like. They struggle inwardly with the impulse to touch him and miss the perfect opportunity to convey their interest.

If you are finding it difficult to touch a guy you like, here are some ways you can break the touch barrier.

- When you are meeting him for a date, come from behind him and gently rest your hand on his shoulders. Let your hand linger on his shoulder for two to three seconds before taking them off. He will replay the sensation of the touch over and over in his mind.

- When you laugh during your conversation, seize that opportunity to touch his arm or shoulder. Let your hand linger a little while before taking it off.

- When you are taking a walk, stop abruptly and when he looks back at you, look at your hands and say, "Well, this hand isn't going to hold itself!" He will take your hand in his and continue the walk.

- "Accidentally" miss your step when you are with him. He will have his hand all over you trying to save his damsel in distress.

- You can save the touch till you say goodbye. Touching his forearm as you walk away or lightly brushing your lips against his cheek as you whisper in his ears, "See you around," will leave him wanting to see you again.

Where to Touch Him

A soft touch on his forearm, waist, shoulders, and the side of his face will clearly convey romantic interests. But be careful with the shoulders. If you pat or squeeze his shoulders he may begin to think of you as a concerned friend.

You can take touching up a notch by kissing him on his cheek. It should be a deliberate short and quick grazing of his skin with your lips, not a sloppy or wet kiss. Another flirtatious move is to give him a gentle kick under the table. Since no one knows what you are doing except him, it sends him a very personal message. But I strongly suggest that you use this type of touch only when you have known each other a little bit more. Using it during a first meeting can be interpreted as desperation.

Keep an Open Body Language

Directly face the guy you are flirting with. Use hand gestures (within reason) to emphasize your words. Place your hands together in your lap when listening to your man. These are all ways your body language can convey openness. On the other hand, certain body postures unconsciously tell people that you are unapproachable. Crossing your arms and slumping (having a drooping posture) will discourage people from coming to you.

Moving Your Body

The following body movements can be made into flirtatious movements.

- Swaying your hips while you walk toward or away from your target. It calls his attention to your hips. Also, sticking your hips sideways while standing close to him draws his attention to the way your hip is provocatively positioned.

- Leaning toward him while sitting close to him tells him you are comfortable with him.

- Ostentatiously crossing and un-crossing your legs calls his attention to your hot legs.

How to Correctly Flirt With Body Movement

Straighten your spine. Mentally feel the sensations at the tail of your spine and in your crotch. Connect with that feeling and let it dictate how your body responds. Instead of being mechanical with your movements, ask yourself, "What does my body want right now?" Is it sex, fun, romance, or what? Let your mind loose and your imagination to run wild. Then get up and walk, flip your hair, lean in closer, or do whatever it is that comes naturally.

If you continue to check in with how you feel as you interact with your target, you will take your flirting body language to a deeper level. Flirting will be a more meaningful experience for you. This method may sound strange to many women, but the truth is that if you are suppressing a sexual feeling within you, you are not likely to seamlessly sway your hips or use any of the other body movements in a way that will send a powerful subliminal message to a man. When you disconnect with your sexual feelings, you may be doing all the right moves, but that will just be putting up an act. The people around you can subconsciously pick up the negative energy you are giving off. Instead of attracting them, they will see through your act and become disinterested.

So go ahead. Permit yourself to mentally check in with what your body is saying. If your crotch is not excited and you are not feeling any sexual sensations in your body, discontinue flirting until the feeling returns.

Other Flirting Signals

Here are some other things you can do to flirt with a guy you like.

1. Change where you are sitting or standing to a place that will encourage him to approach you. This is useful if you sense he is uncomfortable approaching you when you are with other people.

2. Walk past him and seductively look back over your shoulder at him.

3. Slightly tilt your head while gazing into his eyes.

4. Touch your necklace once or twice to draw his attention to your neckline.

5. Smile at him and beckon him with your index finger to come closer.

6. If you are dancing together, get really close to him but don't touch him.

7. Part your lips slightly while giving him a sexy look.

8. Pretend to be shy when you smile at his compliments.

9. Look at his lips for a little longer than normal.

10. Compliment him.

Flirting: The Breakdown

It is better to do what comes naturally when it comes to flirting. But consider the following as a general guide to flirting, especially if the concept is alien to you. It is a simple rundown of how to combine body language and flirtatious words to get a man's attention.

1. **Spot your target**: This is the easy part. You see him at a bar, party, an event, or a mutual friend introduced him and you like him. He could be someone you've had a crush on from work, school, or your neighborhood. And he could be a total stranger. Whichever is the case, if you spot him and you like him, he is your target. Go for the kill! Embrace your feelings for him and flow with what

your body is telling you. Going for the kill simply means calling his attention and making it look like he's the one going for the kill. We are women, and that is something we are naturally good at. The next steps are ways to call his attention.

2. **Make eye contact**: Use your eyes to draw his attention as described above. If he likes what he sees, he will hold your gaze or wait for you to look at him again. A clear indication that he is interested is if he smiles at you while holding your gaze. Once you get his attention, use any of the body language described above to confirm your message to him. For example, you could do the hair flip, play with your hair, slightly bite your lips, or run slowly your hand from your neck down your shoulders and across your body. Alternatively, and if you are feeling generous, you could send him a refill on whatever drink he is having.

3. **Close the gap**: At this point, men will generally want to come closer to you. You have the chance to add verbal flirting to body language at this point. But if he doesn't come to you, you can be more daring and walk up to him. You can use the excuse of looking at something such as a piece of artwork, framed photograph, or anything near him to get closer to him. Alternatively (and I love this tactic),

walk directly past him and pause a few feet away from him. Then look over your shoulder as if something suddenly caught your attention. Don't turn around, just walk backward and say, "Hi handsome. Is this seat taken?" He will most likely be impressed by your audacity and smooth delivery.

4. **Start a conversation**: Once both of you are within earshot, either of you will naturally start talking. But if he is the shy type, he will probably want you to take the lead. If he is a total stranger, you can make small talks. Keep gazing into his eyes while smiling. It will encourage him to keep the conversation going. If he was introduced by a mutual friend, you could continue talking with him from that point, after all, he is already within earshot. Let your conversation be lively. You could say a few jokes or laugh heartily at his jokes.

5. **Flirt with him**: Use one or more flirting body language to communicate your interest to him. If he was not sure you were flirting with him, this is the point to drive home the message. It doesn't mean you should come off strong as someone desperate. What you should do at this point is to give him the chance to chase after you.

6. **Gauge his response**: Try to gauge the level of his interest. Is he smiling back at you? Is he speaking animatedly? Does he seem distracted or seem to be expecting someone else? Is he bored or giving his attention to his phone? Is he encouraging you to be more forthcoming? Figuring out these things can help you continue flirting or call it off.

7. **Exchange numbers (optional)**: If you feel comfortable with his level of interest and would like to contact him again, you could ask for his contact details. It is okay to ask him first. Many men are intrigued by women who take the initiative in such situations. You can choose to leave this out if you don't want to contact him again, if you are just out to have a good time teasing men, or if you are just practicing to improve your flirting skills.

8. **Initiate tactile touch (optional)**: You could go ahead and touch him to convey your interest as I've described earlier.

9. **Know when to walk away (very important)**: Perhaps this is the most important aspect of flirting. If you overstay your welcome, your interaction can become boring one or he may

begin to see you as a desperate woman. But it doesn't mean you should run away either, even if the man shows little or no interest. Always leave an interaction on a positive note, regardless of whatever happens. If the conversation is not as you expected, simply smile at him, say goodbye, and walk away. Keep in mind that not all interactions will lead to attraction. On the other hand, if he seems to enjoy what you are doing and saying, you can still cut it short and walk away leaving him longing for more. You could do that after exchanging contact details (if you want) and then touch him softly while saying goodbye.

Knowing The Right Situation For Flirting

Flirting doesn't work in all situations. Your timing has to be right to create any sort of impact on your target. For example, the workplace may not be the perfect place to flirt even if you think a coworker might be interested in you. Moreover, many organizations do not encourage their employees to enter into romantic relationships. It is also possible that your actions will be interpreted as sexual harassment.

Do keep in mind also that the cute guy behind the counter is paid to be courteous. So, when you interact with him as a customer, make sure not to confuse his friendly gesture to mean that he is flirting back at you. He is most likely just doing his job.

A more suitable situation for flirting would be outside work or business environment such as during parties and at social events. After hours are great times for flirting. You could go to a bar or club where you are sure your crush visits regularly. And even if you don't have a particular man in mind, hang out in places where guys spend time and you are likely to spot one to flirt with. Before you walk up to a guy, make sure you have observed him long enough to determine that he is alone and not waiting for a potential partner. It would be awkward trying to start a conversation with a man you find attractive only for his woman to show up.

Chapter 6

The Art of Seduction

First Things First

Before you jump into seducing a man, the following few things need to be put in the right perspective.

What's Your Reason?

One huge obstacle to seduction is doing it to prove a point to yourself or make you feel better about yourself. That is completely backward. You should feel good about yourself and develop the right mindset (as we've seen in previous chapters) before attempting to seduce any man. You need to define exactly what your reason is for seducing anyone and that reason shouldn't be to make you feel good about yourself. For example, if you think you are unattractive but seducing an attractive guy would prove that you are attractive after all, it means your underlying reason is twisted to begin with. You are placing the cart before the horse. Work on improving your self-esteem first before seducing anyone, not the other way round.

Here's the main reason it is a bad idea to try to prove your self-worth with seduction. You are not going to be yourself in the seduction. You are merely putting up an act, and you will be very careful not to make a mistake because your self-worth is hanging in the balance. In other words, you are acting like a seductress, but you truly are not one. Your words and actions will be borne out of desperation. It is similar to someone who is trying too hard to be funny when they are not. Their words and actions end up being awkward. But someone who is naturally funny doesn't bother or think too hard about being funny. They are carefree about how they behave and are funny in the process even when they are not making any effort to be funny.

To be successful at seduction, you must begin to see the world from the viewpoint of a seductress and change your mentality to that of a seductress—a carefree embrace of your sexuality—and then combine that with the right seductive moves. And the way to go about developing the mindset of a seductress is to first get clear on why you want to seduce a guy.

Are you looking for a man who will commit to an exclusive loving relationship? Are you just interested in a casual hookup? Are you trying to make a man fall in love with you? Are you trying to be more than a friend to a man who thinks of you as just a friend? Are you interested in the excitement of the chase? It doesn't matter what your goal for wanting to seduce a man is, as long as it is not to prove a point, you are fine. Once you have defined your goal, the next step is to not bother about the outcome.

Enjoy the Process Regardless of the Outcome

Becoming obsessed about one particular guy and believing that somehow your fantasy about him will materialize is likely to put you under undue pressure to make things work between you and him. Instead of having fun and enjoying the art of seduction, you will become worried and fearful that your dream may not come true. Fear and worry can diminish your chances of success.

Before you start to seduce a man, make up your mind that you are going to thoroughly enjoy yourself and not bother your pretty head over what ought, might, should or shouldn't have been. Fun should be your watchword, not fear or worry.

To think and feel like a seductress, you must let go of the need to have a particular outcome. A true seductress doesn't think that her happiness depends on one particular man. Neither does she thinks that being with a particular guy will make her life complete. This frees her from being clingy. She doesn't build a fantasy and try to coerce reality to suit the dream in her head. She simply has fun in the moments she interacts with her man and let things happen naturally.

Have More than One Option

Indeed, we have the ability to attract the man we want. (Oh, and it feels so good to have the one we desire.) But it doesn't always happen that way. Sometimes, he is taken, not interested in us, or not ready to be in a relationship. If you put all your eggs in one basket and fixate on only one guy, you could be headed for some major heartbreak. Keep your options open. Apart from improving your seduction skills, it also:

- Puts you in the position to choose from several other desirable options. You don't have to wait indefinitely until one particular guy thinks you are worthy of his time and affection. You are not at the mercy of any guy.

- Removes any form of obsession over any particular man.

- Reminds you that you don't have to put up with someone who clearly isn't interested in you or living up to your expectations.

- Tells him that if he truly wants to have you all to himself in an exclusive relationship, he will need to make that very clear without you needing to push him to do so.

Okay, so now that we have covered some ground rules, let us see how you can seduce a man to come after you as if his life depends on it.

How to Make Him Chase After You Indefinitely

Seduction without charm, as I've mentioned before, is a pathetic display of desperation. Seducing a man should be what you do after you have attracted him to you and not before. Charm and flirt with him to get his attention. Use seduction to strengthen the "magnetic" pull you have over him. In this section, I'll take you through five important lessons on the art of seducing a man. Learn and apply these lessons to get the man of your dreams chasing after you.

Unpredictability

In Chapter 2, I mentioned that men tend to be analytical and logical. In other words, men tend to want to figure things out. They are generally more pattern-seeking than us. But that in itself is a problem because as soon as they have something figured out, it becomes boring to them. Therefore, this is your first lesson in the art of seduction: **be unpredictable**. One-dimensional characters are not interested whether in movies or in real-life. They don't hold anyone's attention for long. The same applies to men and their desires for women. Once it becomes predictable or one-dimensional—as soon as they have you all figured out—they lose interest and the chase ends.

To remain interesting for your man means that you are unpredictable. Men are intrigued by women who are full of paradoxes, mysteries, and are generally hard to decode. I am not suggesting that you should create some sort of fake complexity about your persona; that would mean living a lie. You need to be yourself and enjoy being so. Being unpredictable is certainly not about playing hard to get, but it is about breaking your patterns. Just when a guy thinks he's got you all figured out, you do something out of character and blow him away.

To a man, being unpredictable and interesting means:

1. Suggesting something he would never expect from you.

2. Keeping him guessing what your next move would be. Never let him know every one of your moves before you make them.

3. Trying out some of his sexual fantasies when he least expects it. If you are already having sex with a guy, it is easy to become predictable. Up your game by trying any of the following:

    - Do some crazy bedroom moves.
    - Leave the lights on if you are used to having sex in a dimly light room or total darkness.
    - Put your hands in his pants and fondle him in an elevator, taxi, or any public place where you risk being seen.

4. Taking time to know random facts about different things. The more knowledgeable you are the better you can hold intellectual conversations with him on things that he least expect you to know anything about. Beauty and brains are the perfect attraction for a man.

5. Get him to talk more about himself instead of revealing too much about yourself. Disclose as

little information about yourself as you can and keep him digging for more.

6. Being independent even when you are in a relationship with him. Have and pursue your interest. It is a huge turn-on for men.

7. Having fun without him. Being able to chat, laugh, and have a good time with friends when he's busy with his friends is good for your mental and emotional health. And it makes him know your happiness doesn't depend on him.

8. Change your routine every once in a while. Call, text, or chat with him at different times.

9. Standing or sitting close to him yet avoiding physical touch even when it is obvious that you should touch, kiss, or hug him. Let your touch not follow a predictable pattern or timing. You can lean in as if to kiss him, linger for a few seconds, and pull back.

10. Be adventurous. Explore different places. Branch out of your usual route and learn things about a completely different culture.

Psychology

The second lesson in the art of seduction is this: ***seduction is more about psychology than beauty***. What this comes down to is pretty simple. To seduce a man, you don't have to look like a movie star or that hot model on the cover of a magazine. Those images on the cover of magazines and TV are a product of professional photographers, editors, pre- and-post-production crews, and a host of others. Stop trying to look like people that don't exist in real life because even the models don't look anything like the people on the media.

Every woman who puts her mind to it can become great at seduction because, by nature, a woman is designed to seduce. All you need is to begin to see the world through the eyes of a seducer. This means you need to first define what is it you want to achieve (getting a man hooked to you, attracting him sexually, or making him do what you want). Next is to know what actions to take to penetrate the defenses of your target—in this case, your target is the man. What are his likes and dislikes? Is he on social media? Does he get to read his texts, chats, and emails? Or does he prefer phone calls?

Of course, you don't have to know every detail about a man, especially if you have not known him for too long. However, within a couple of minutes interacting with a man or certainly after a few dates, you should be able to deduce a handful of useful information that can help you penetrate his defenses. Remember that if you have correctly flirted with him and have drawn his attention to you, he is probably beginning to be attracted to you. This means your job of seduction is a lot easier. He already finds you likable so when he sees the efforts you expend on his behalf to get him sexually interested in you or to get him to know that you care about him and how much he is worth to you, it increases his attraction and likeness for you.

Create Temptation

The third thing you need to know about the art of seduction is this: ***tempt your man to awaken a desire in him which he cannot control***. Find his weakness and fantasy then give him a hint (through words or action) that suggests that you can make his dream come true. Try to find out his definition of romance, his sexual fantasies, and so on. He will usually signal some of his weaknesses and fantasies in casual comments and little details that elude his conscious control.

Entice him by dropping elusive hints and innuendoes laden with sexual connotations. Be suggestive both in words and actions. He'll not be able to place a finger on exactly what you are saying or doing, yet he knows there's some other meaning to your words and actions. This keeps the attraction going.

To make the temptation stronger, take him beyond his psychological limit to explore what he considers forbidden or taboo. When you stir up in him a sense of transgression, it makes the temptation stronger. If what you are tempting him with is normal and ordinary, it won't make him feel he is yielding to his "dark side." Understand that men secretly desire to explore their so-called dark sides. He will seek you out to "lead him into temptation!"

Suspense

Most people hardly find a movie interesting after a spoiler. The suspense and enjoyment are removed after a spoiler. The same applies to seduction which makes the fourth lesson in the art of seduction thus: *always keep your man in suspense*. Let your man keep wondering what you are up to. If he can read you, you will need to break your pattern as earlier discussed in the first lesson in the art of seduction. The less predictable you become, the higher the sense of suspense you can create in him.

Pleasure and Pain

The fifth and final lesson in the art of seduction is this: ***always mix pleasure with pain***. I do not mean that you should inflict physical pain on your man. If your seduction offers pleasure on a straight path toward a climax without a twist along the way, the climax will come too soon and the pleasure will be weak. To make him feel the pleasure more intensely, introduce a sense of pain, suffering, or deprivation during seduction. Suffering and pain will increase his appreciation for the pleasure he gets at the end. Begin your seduction by luring him in a particular direction, then when his expectation is high, change course and appear uninterested. This is the perfect setup for maneuvering him however you want. But be sure that whatever it is you want him to do is in line with his character or else you risk ruining your perfect setup.

A Few Seductive Ideas

I am quite sure by now you have several scenarios running through your mind and what seductive things you will do to your man. But just in case you are still finding it hard to come up with something 100% original, let me share a few simple ideas that can help you seduce him. Remember to put your spin on it and make it your own idea.

- Bring him along when shopping for new lingerie. Let him watch you try on different sexy lingerie. He will be dying to touch you but simply can't.

- Go about your house chores without panties and make sure he knows you are not wearing anything under.

- Play a nice and slow sensual song. Turn off the lights in your bedroom, and light just one candle. The soft dim glow of the candle will light up his passion.

- Take his hand and use it to slowly touch your body the way you want and where you want him to touch you.

- While he is in the shower, put on a white t-shirt and nothing else, then go ahead and join him in the shower.

- Take a picture of your bare legs in the new heels you just bought and send it to his phone while he is at work.

- Answer the door barely clothed. Be sure he's the one at the door to avoid awkward moments with someone else.

- When you are really horny, touch yourself while he watches.

- One night when he least expects it, wear only thigh-highs and climb into bed. He'll take it from there.

- Take off your bra while he watches, and then return to what you were doing. He'll keep thinking of those lovely breasts and wanting to hold them.

- During sex, tell him how big and hard he is. Tell him how good he is in bed. Tell him how wet you are and how you like what he is doing. It will turn him on more. Don't be the hush-hush type in bed. Be careful not to tell him things he knows are lies.

- Take off your panties, sit from across him where he can have a good view of you and "accidentally" give him a flash when you cross or un-cross your legs.

- Spray a fragrant perfume all over your hair and tie it up into a ponytail. When he is standing or sitting next to you, let down your hair and let the sweet smell of your hair work its magic.

- During foreplay, instruct him to figure out a way to enjoy your sexy body without using his hands. You'll be amazed at how creative he can be.

- Put on your bikini and ask him if it still fits.

- Initiate foreplay, get him really in the mood and then walk away. He'll crave you like crazy!

- Slip out of your panties and pass it to him under the dining table.

- Lightly bite your lower lip, wink at him, and walk away. If you go to the bedroom or where you will be alone, he'll likely come after you.

Using the Right Seductive Words and Texts

You don't have to be physically present with a man to seduce him. You can leave notes, call him on his mobile phone, or send him text messages. Whatever you do, remember that seductive texts or calls are not the same as phone sex. So, try not to send him any of your nude pictures or clips. The idea is to make him yearn to be with you and not to bare everything on his phone. Also, remember to adapt the following texts and questions to suit your particular situation. Using them verbatim may come across as unnatural and cold. In all, keep it playful, witty, and don't bother your brains too much about sending the perfect text or using the right words.

Seductive Texts

Here are some ideas for seductive text messages.

1. Send him this when you are at work, "I can't focus on work. All I can think of is you on my bed... naked."

2. Send this to him, right after he leaves for work, "Something hot and steamy awaits you tonight!"

3. Send this to him very early in the morning, "Guess what we did in my dreams last night..."

4. Send this to him just before you sleep, "I'll be waiting for you tonight... in my dreams."

5. Send him a picture of a sexy bra and ask, "Do you think this will fit?"

6. Send him a picture of your hot legs and say, "I'm not wearing any undies... wanna see?"

7. Send him a picture of a lollipop and say, "I like the way this lollipop feels on my tongue and lips. It

reminds me of something about you. Can you guess?"

8. On a cold night, send him this, "If you were here right now…"

9. The next day after spending the night in your place, send him this text, "My sheets still smell of you!"

10. If he's out of town for a couple of days, send him this, "I miss having your hands all over my body, ripping off my flimsy panties and doing filthy things to me."

Dirty Questions

You can put a twist to your dirty talk. Instead of just talking dirty, ask him dirty questions such as the ones below:

1. "Do you think this tattoo/birthmark on my thigh/boobs is sexy?" Ask this while showing him the tattoo or birthmark wherever it is on your body. Skip this if you don't have any.

2. "I'm getting some lessons on giving a massage. Can I practice on you?" You don't have to know how to give a perfect massage before you use this.

3. Whisper this question in his ears, "What that thing you would like to try with me but haven't had the guts to ask?"

4. "What's the craziest thing you've ever done sexually?" You can use this question to set the mood for a sensual evening with him.

5. Lay your head on his laps and ask, "What is the wildest sexual fantasy you've ever had?"

6. Pull your dress to reveal you cleavage, wink and ask, "If I only had two choices; to work as a stripper or porn star, which would you want me to choose and why?"

Whether it leads to sex or not, the mere act of seducing him through your actions, words, and texts will keep him thinking about you even when you're not with him. The important thing is to be bold enough to express the sexual feelings you feel inside of you. You cannot suppress your sexuality and expect someone else to feel what you don't want to feel.

Chapter 7

Personal Grooming

Personal grooming is not vanity. It is a necessity for every woman who wants to be appreciated the way she is. Personal grooming is about accepting your body as it is and then making every part of it have the best appeal and appearance possible. This does not necessarily mean wearing designer labels or applying a ton of makeup. Even if you are a model, you don't live your life on the runway or the red carpet.

However, don't mistake looking gorgeous for being attractive. It is easy for women to assume that men are more attracted to the most gorgeous looking lady in the room. Not true! Men are more attracted to positive attitudes than great looks. Of course, the woman with the gorgeous look is likely to draw quick attention to herself but if she lacks a great attitude, she'll push the men away as quickly as she can get their attention. The perfect combo would be to appear gorgeous and also have a great attitude.

But personal grooming is just about what you wear, how your face looks and how glowing your skin is. It is all of that and how a woman carries herself, especially in public. You can't possibly make any man find you attractive if you draw his attention with your beauty and then start picking your nose in public or some other gross unladylike behavior for goodness sake. This chapter will focus on how to take care of your physical appearance, how to carry yourself elegantly, and how to break free from any self-limiting beliefs.

Your Physical Appearance Matters

No man in his right senses will find you attractive if your hair is untidy, your face is smeared in makeup, your fingernails are dirty, and your clothes are rumpled. Flirting when you are unkempt is very creepy. Your first order of business as a woman who intends to be flirty is personal grooming. And here are some great tips to help you with that.

Your Skin is Your Top Priority

Your skin is the largest organ in your entire body and is what people first see when they come in contact with you. You should definitely give it adequate care and attention. It doesn't matter how great your liver, pancreas, heart, or any other internal organs are, no one sees them, not even you. If your biggest external organ (your skin) isn't healthy and glowing, it would be difficult to get anyone interested in your healthy lungs.

Every woman should be best friends with her mirror. It tells you what your skin looks like—not just your face. When you stand in front of your mirror, look at the skin on your entire body; face, neck, chest, arms, elbows, trunk, belly, waist, thigh, legs, and feet. Obsessing about your face and neglecting the rest of your body is not proper care of your skin.

Make sure you bathe regularly and use an exfoliating body scrub. There are countless types of moisturizers in the market; select the ones that suit your skin type and remember to moisturize your knees, elbows, and feet. During winter or cold seasons, keep your skin well moisturized to avoid chapped skin. Sunscreens can also help to protect your delicate skin from harmful rays. Develop the habit of washing your face at least two times daily with a mild face wash. Whatever makeup you apply, make sure you wash it off before you go to bed at night. Also, remember that cosmetics have expiration dates. Don't just continue to use a cosmetic because it is still available; make it a habit to note the expiration date of each of your cosmetics and get new ones long before they expire.

Besides beauty products, you can also help to keep your skin healthy and glowing by drinking lots of water and eating healthily. As a matter of fact, this is the healthiest option for maintaining healthy and glowing skin. This is what makes your beauty shine from within. Consider including fruits and green vegetables in your daily meals. Make physical exercises a part of your daily routine. You don't need to have a goal of losing weight before you start working out. Exercising regularly (at least 4 to 5 times a week) can help to keep your skin reenergized. Also, make sure to get adequate and quality sleep every night (at least seven to eight hours of sleep) to help rejuvenate your skin.

Use Makeup Sensibly

Pick eyeliners, eye shadows, and mascaras that suit your eyes. Choose facial products—foundation, concealer, face powder, and so on that are safe for your face. Mineral-based products are always better as they are less prone to cause skin irritation. This is not to teach you how to use your makeup, but there aren't many men who would like to encounter a baked face.

Remember that makeup is meant to complement your look and not to completely change your entire self.

Some ladies would prefer to not use makeup, and that is okay. Celebrities such as Alicia Keys, Ellen Page, Demi Lovato, Shailene Woodley, and Gigi Hadid are known to have either completely ditched makeup or use it less frequently, yet they still look fabulous. So, it doesn't matter whether you want your face to have as much makeup as that of Katie Price or as little or no makeup as that of Jessica Alba, the important thing to keep in mind is to do what suits your face, mood and dress.

Whether you use makeup or not, make sure that your lips are not scaly. Use a lip balm, lipstick, lip gloss or whatever you prefer to soothe your lips and keep them moist and succulent. As a woman who intends to flirt, let your lips give a man something to think about, if you know what I mean.

Always Carry the Essentials

As a lady, you shouldn't leave home without having your essentials handy. Consider it as your survival kit that can help you quickly fix any blemish when you are out of your house. Your survival kit could be a Ziploc bag containing items for your nails, hair, skin, and so on. Some of the essentials you can put inside your survival kit include:

- Compact towel
- Mints (very essential)
- Hairbands
- Vaseline or lotion
- Mini comb
- Mini mirror
- Miniature sewing kit
- Perfume or cologne
- Pins

Remember that going out of your house for a date, to the workplace, or for shopping is not the same as going on a trip or camping. So, keep the contents of your survival kit to only essential stuff you most definitely need.

Maintain Your Hairstyle

If you cannot maintain long hair, cut it. Your hairstyle should suit your face to accentuate your beautiful face. Wearing the wrong hairstyle can mar your outlook. Remember to wash your hair regularly with shampoo and conditioner. Also, nourish your hair with good hair oil. If you keep long hair, you could choose to tie it up into a high ponytail or in a neat bun. This is particularly a useful style to use when you want to expose your neck—a spot the male folks find attractive. Hair sprays and gels may be harmful to your hair texture. If you want to use them, make sure that they are safe for your hair. Here is one unforgivable blunder you must avoid at all costs especially in public, never be caught scratching your head in public.

Remove Unwanted Hair

Shave off lip hair, if you have any. You may also want to remove hair from your upper arm and thighs if you have naturally long and dark body hair. Keep your eyebrows neat also.

Regularly remove armpit hair as well as pubic hair. But if you are a woman who thinks that pubic hair is sexy, go ahead and keep it. Just make sure it is always neat. However, consider trimming it at the bikini line if you intend to go to a beach. Whether you choose to remove your pubic hair is entirely up to you. There has been a recent trend encouraging women not to shave their pubic hair. Women want to make the decision to shave or not based on personal choices and not societal pressure. Whichever side of the divide you fall, just make sure you are neat down there. Hopefully, before you go to bed with the man of your dreams, you'll have figured out whether or not pubic hair disgusts him.

Dress Sensibly

Always wear comfortable clothing that makes you feel confident and accentuate your curves. No man wants to date their grandma. Nevertheless, tight-fitting clothes, see-through dresses, or miniskirt that barely covers your butt is likely to convey a message that says you are trying too hard to get noticed. Wear fresh, clean clothes that are properly ironed and appropriate for a particular place and occasion. If you are going into a professional setting (work, business meeting, and so on), play down on your jewelry to avoid drawing unnecessary attention to yourself. Put on footwear that is very comfortable for you. People may not have ulterior motives for looking at your footwear, but when they do, it gives them an impression about you.

De-pill Your Clothes

Some types of clothes can have their threads and fibers come off like little balls after a while. These build-up of fiber balls called pilling can make your clothes look old and worn out. De-pilling your clothes doesn't require any special equipment. Use a sharp razor to gently shave off the pilling making sure that you are slow while shaving off the threads and fibers to avoid putting holes in your dress.

Smell Nice

If your scent hits the people that come in contact with you, then you should consider toning down that strong scent. A woman's scent should remind the people of flowers and fruits. A gentle, soft, and light smell that lingers is better than a harsh and strong smell that feels heavy and jarring to the nose.

Keep Your Nails Clean and Take Care of Your Teeth

Whether you like long or short nails, make sure they are clean. Both your hand and toenails should look attractive and trimmed.

Brush your teeth and floss regularly. Apart from having mints handy, keep your appointments with your dentist to avoid cavities or bad breath.

Be Polite

It doesn't take away anything from you to be polite. Saying "please," "thank you," and "sorry," shows how well cultured and courteous you are. While it is good to be open and honest, it is equally good to use friendly and polite words that portray you as intelligent and friendly instead of harsh and insensitive.

Be Graceful

Besides good looks, how you carry yourself when walking, sitting, talking, and your general body posture is equally important. Let your movements be elegant and ladylike. Keep your head up and your shoulders and back straight when walking or sitting. Own your space when you stand by placing your hands on your hips with your legs slightly apart.

A Lasting First Impression

Having the perfect skin, looks, dress, and self-composure are great. Putting these into proper use to make a good and lasting first impression on a guy is even better. I'll share some great tips that can help you turn your dating experience from a nerve-wracking experience (despite your proper grooming) to an interesting experience that makes men come back for you over and over again.

1. **Turn your first date into an event**: Do something unconventional (not crazy) on your first date. Instead of sitting down and making

small talk (that is full of guesswork and may not have a natural flow to it), you can spend a few minutes sitting and chatting before getting active. Go to the park, take a walk, or do just anything besides just sitting down and throwing questions back and forth. Being active can reveal the spontaneous side of both of you, and you'll enjoy the date more than just sitting and doing the traditional chit-chat and eating out.

2. **Express appreciation**: Saying "thank you" seems inconsequential when you are out on a date with a guy. After all, he is supposed to do you favors, please, you, and woo you right? Wrong! Men are protective of their money and are always on the lookout for a gold-digger especially on the first dates. When he picks you up, say thank you. When he opens the door or pulls out a chair for you, say thank you. Thank him for a lovely time, dinner, coffee or whatever it was he bought you on your date. Showing your appreciation will remove any concern he has about you being a gold-digger or one of those unappreciative ladies.

3. **Maintaining eye contact**: Look into his eyes when he's talking to you. Since you're not trying to stare him down, make sure you have a smile dancing on the corner of your lips while you are

looking at him. Even if you are the shy type, make sure to keep your eyes on his other facial features but mostly on his eyes. You'll make the connection between you stronger by maintaining eye contact. If he is talking to you and a waiter or waitress comes along, keep your eyes on his and let him finish before you take your eyes off him and begin ordering. You're subliminally telling him that he is the most important person in your world at that moment. He will get the message and will most likely treat and respect you in the same way.

4. **Smile**: A smile says you are relaxed, open, welcoming, and it encourages your date to be more open to you too. Besides, guys find you more attractive when you smile and it can also lead to moments of hearty laughter together—moments he will play over and over again in his mind when he thinks back on your outing together.

5. **Be mysterious**: It's a date, not an inquisition. You don't have to recount the entire story of your life to him. You are likely to bore him by revealing too much too soon. And it also spoils the fun of discovering who you are. You are depriving him of finding out by himself the mystery of who you are by laying everything bare for him. Even if you tend to be talkative, keep your responses brief so that

you don't run him over with too much talk. Instead of telling him everything about yourself, you can simply focus on the details of a few things.

6. **Show less skin**: Wearing a dress that reveals too much skin—legs, cleavage, or even your sexy flat belly—can become a distraction to the man, especially on your first date. Dress to cover your body properly, unless you are only interested in getting laid and getting him to think a lot about sex throughout your date. Save yourself the headache of trying to show him too much skin; there's a huge chance that he is already mentally stripping you. That may sound creepy to you, but that's just how men are wired. They don't need to see excess skin to visualize us naked. So, don't spoil the fun for him. However, here's something classy you could do to help him see your curves differently. If you wore a skirt on your first date, switch to jeans on the second date or put on a nice fitting skirt on the second date if you wore jeans on the first date. This will present your delicate curves to him in a new light.

7. **Switch off your phone**: Yes, turn your phone off. I am not saying put it on silent, don't text while on a date, or don't take calls. I am saying switch off your phone. That way you will not be tempted to

even look at it and it tells the man how much you value your time together. To make this more effective, make him know you are turning off your phone. Say something like, "Just a minute please let me put my phone off so we can have this moment to ourselves!" Put your phone off and continue by saying, "So, you were saying?" He will get the message loud and clear and he will distinguish you from all the other dates he had ever been on.

8. **No dramas, please**: Keep your conversation positive at all times, especially on your first date. If you had a bad day, if your ex was a jerk, or whatever negative things are happening or have happened, please keep them completely out of your conversation with your date. Remember, you are on a date to figure out if it could lead to something good between you two. It is not a conversation with your best friend, your gossip mate, your mom, or your husband. Avoid dumping negative stuff on him. You'll simply drive him away.

9. **Stop trying too hard**: It is a good idea to put your best foot forward on your first date but make sure you remain interesting instead of trying too hard to impress him. Only mention the things you

are good at if mentioning them would score you some good points. However, be tactful when mentioning it. You could cleverly steer the conversation in that direction or seize the opportunity if he happens to mention something related to it. Alternatively, you could make him talk about something he is passionate about. For example, if you have noticed on his social media page that he loves swimming, you could casually mention something related to swimming and watch how he comes alive with excitement. Keep him going with encouraging nods and looking deep into his eyes as he talks about his passion. He will want to share more moments with the woman that lights him up.

Self-Limiting Beliefs and How to Overcome Them

Every woman is capable of attracting a man. We are genetically engineered to do just that. But some of us have allowed ourselves to buy into erroneous assumptions and perceptions about ourselves and how the world works. The way to know these assumptions are self-limiting is when they begin to hold you back from what you are capable of achieving.

Some of these assumptions are:

- I am too old to start flirting.

- No man will be interested in someone like me.

- I don't have enough experience with men.

- I am not gorgeous enough.

- Other ladies are better than me.

- I'm afraid I'm going to get hurt.

- I need to become a different person to deserve the man I want.

- I am too young. Older ladies will snatch him from me.

- It is selfish to want a man all to myself.

- A woman shouldn't make the first move.

- Men are cheats. I can't trust them.

- True love is very rare.

- I am not really good at maintaining relationships.

- What is destined to happen will happen whether or not I make an effort.

The more you think such thoughts and add emotions to them (feel that they are true), the stronger these patterns of thinking become inside your brain. Neural pathways inside your brain are strengthened to support these thinking patterns. Remember that your mind doesn't know whether something you believe is true or not. If you continue to supply the data, it will accept it as true and begin to selectively sift through your experiences to filter out things that support your belief.

Self-Limiting Beliefs Become Self-Fulfilling Prophecies

Once your mind accepts a belief as true, that belief becomes a self-fulfilling prophecy. Self-limiting beliefs are unhealthy beliefs and will definitely lead you into unhealthy behaviors and habits. And herein lies the self-fulfilling prophecy cycle. Unhealthy behaviors as a result of unhealthy beliefs will head to negative outcomes. The negative outcomes then reinforce the unhealthy (self-limiting) beliefs. This can become a vicious cycle that is very tough to break.

For example, a woman has a strong belief that she is unlovable because she grew up in a family where her parents didn't show her much love. She goes from one relationship to another with that belief and she gets hurt over and over again. The men she dated treated her exactly as she had expected, which is very poorly. Her experience with dating and relationships reinforces her belief that she is unlovable.

But what she failed to see is that her beliefs are stopping her from doing things differently. She approached every man and every relationship with the same expectation and got exactly what she expected. Her core beliefs are stopping her from taking steps to improve herself. No man will love you if you don't love yourself enough to improve your habits and behaviors.

Overcoming Self-Limiting Beliefs

As a woman, you must be open and honest with yourself the beliefs you hold regarding your looks, sexuality, sensuality, and all the sexual and relationship taboos you grew up believing. Until you can confront these beliefs and challenge their origins and then determine whether they serve you or hinder you, you may find yourself unable to enjoy your sexual relationships to the max.

It is in a bid to effectively combat and overcome these beliefs that I shared the exercises in Chapter 1. If you find yourself doubting your capability to be flirt or seduce any man of your choice, I encourage you to put these exercises into practice until you feel the exhilaration and freedom that comes from totally accepting yourself the way you are. Note that the man you flirt with may not necessarily become interested in you sexually. This is why I earlier stated that flirting is not just something that you do to someone; instead, it is about how you connect and accept your sensuality and sexuality. In other words, whether or not a man becomes interested in you, your self-esteem improves with each flirting experience you have. The better you feel about yourself the greater your chances of getting rid of self-limiting beliefs and attracting men easily.

Don't Settle for the Bone – Go For the Steak!

One self-limiting belief many women have is that a woman should make the first move to attract a man. First of all, that notion is completely bogus! Consciously or unconsciously, a woman always makes the first move and scientific research supports this (Fisher, 2016). The way we make up, dress up, carry and comport ourselves, conveys a lot of nonverbal signals to men. It tells them whether to come for us or to steer clear of us. We may not even be aware of these signals but we are sending them out anyway. So, yes, we may not deliberately make the first move by walking up to a guy (although some women do that), but we make the first move by sending subtle messages about our willingness to be approached or not.

Whether it is a conscious or unconscious move, you don't have to wait for a man you like to come to you. Don't limit yourself with the faulty reasoning that says the patient dog eats the fattest bone. It doesn't always work that way in attracting men. If you let yourself buy into that belief, you may find yourself asking why all the good men are taken. Dogs don't necessarily prefer bones; they prefer steak but settle for bones in the absence of meat. In finding the man of your dreams, don't settle. Go for what you want. Put the charming, flirting, and seduction techniques you've learned in this book into practice. The more you practice, the better you become. The better you become, the easier it is to attract the man you really desire and deserve.

Chapter 8

What Next?

Yes! He took the bait and fell for you, or at least so you think. Well, what next after the man of your dreams shows interest in you? What if he is attracted to you and even had sex with you? What next? Do you nudge him into a committed relationship or do you let him be? How do you know he is truly head over heels for you or just interested in the sex? What if he wants more than a fling? What if he asks you to be his girlfriend? What if he wants a steady relationship with you? How do you handle all the emotions running through your mind and the excitement you feel all over your body? This chapter will show you exactly what to do next? So, let's begin with whether or not to keep him.

To Keep Him or Not

Ultimately, the decision to continue with a guy after he has indicated interest in you (and maybe even had sex with you) depends largely on why you attracted him in the first place. Were you hoping for just a fling or were you hoping for a long-term relationship? If you are not ready for a committed relationship, it is better to let him know you stand even if he wants more. Be honest and upfront about your decision so that he wouldn't feel you took him for a ride.

If you are a woman who's desperate about getting a man, it may come as a shock to you that some other woman will have a man and not want to keep him. We go through different stages in life and have a wide range of experiences that can be very different from each other even as women. A woman who is divorced or separated may want to explore with different men before deciding whether or not to commit to a relationship again. A young widow may find it difficult to fall in love again, but that doesn't mean she won't find men attractive. It also doesn't mean she is suddenly incapable of having sex and having a good time. A single lady who's never been into any relationship can also choose to explore with different men before making her choice. Whatever your particular situation, if you are not ready to start a committed relationship, don't let one session of passionate sex change your mind. Take your time to get to know your man better while exploring other options. If he is fully aware of your decision to be available to other men and is still interested in you, he will intensify his effort in chasing after you. Perhaps he may get you to change your mind after all.

On the other hand, if you are interested in a long-term relationship, then you should consider making him chase you more. Many women feel they no longer wield any power over a man after they've had sex with him. They assume he has gotten what he wants so they have no more leverage. But this is not true. You are still in charge and can even make him chase you more if you know how to push the right buttons. And here's how to do just that.

1. **Continue looking attractive for other men**: A man wants to earn his prize. A little competition is healthy for your new guy. If he finds that you are still trying to get the attention of other men, he will put in more effort to get you solely to himself. For example, if you post a new sexy picture of yourself on your social media page after you have had a nice time with him, you are telling him that you are still very confident in yourself regardless of

whatever might have happened the previous night. You show him that you are still as hot and flirty as ever and can still be his ultimate fantasy if he has the energy to keep up the chase. If he doesn't, other more capable men will take his place.

2. **Leave out any talk about commitment**: Bring up any talk about commitment too soon (especially right after passionate sex) and you're on the verge of losing your man. Let him move at his pace. If you have sex with a man, enjoy the afterglow. Don't rush out of bed as if you've done something awful. Relax. Be there with him. But leave out any talk about spending the rest of your lives together. And when it is time to go, be the first to get up and get dressed. Don't linger on the bed and try to tell him you don't ever want him to leave your side. Push all such talks and thoughts far away from your mind. It is just your sex hormones pushing you into jeopardizing your budding relationship.

3. **Get him to start the chase all over again**: No matter how long you shy away from sex, you will eventually sleep with him. Whether he falls madly in love with you before the sex or not, it is okay to have sex at some point (unless either or both of

you have decided to be celibate). You need to keep the sparks flying even after sex regardless of whether the sex was too soon or happens much later. Resist the urge to become friends with benefits. If you give him the notion that he can have sex with you anytime he chooses, he'll soon become bored and lose interest in the chase. This is not the same as playing hard to get. Press the reset button, become cordial instead of romantic. It will make him chase you all over again because he wants to feel that connection once again.

4. **Make your next sex better than the first**: Usually, your first sex is based on curiosity and passion. The next time you decide to have sex, find out his sexual fantasies and fulfill as many as you can. Heads up: you're not turning yourself into his sex slave. You are simply blowing his mind and making him have a glimpse into what lays ahead in the future. It will keep the chase going. Of course, you should enjoy as much pleasure as him too. The point is to put in the effort to make subsequent sex a more pleasurable experience for both of you than the first time and to keep improving. If you let sex "happen" as many women do, he'll be quick to find you sexually boring.

5. **Forget about proving your worth**: If a guy who is interested in you, there will be no need to stand on your head or bend over backward just to please him. Going above and beyond to make him happy is an act of desperation and will push him away instead of keeping him glued to you. Being confident and your happy self is both sexy and a turn on for men. Accept that who you are is good enough—there is really no point obsessing over the right things to say to him or do for him. When you relax and be yourself, you tell your man that you have a healthy respect for yourself and your self-confidence is intact. This makes him want you more!

If you find a good man that you intend to keep, be careful of making the following mistakes.

1. **Playing hard to get**: This should be a strategy for getting his attention and should be used for the short-term. But playing hard to get after you've established a connection is a mistake. Don't forget that the chase in the game of flirting has an endpoint beyond which a man wouldn't go. If he has "caught" you as his "prize" (very odd choice of words to use for us women, but I'm sure you get the gist), what you need to focus on is how to keep

him interested, and not how to play hard to get anymore.

2. **Faking unavailability**: There's a huge difference between being available and being clingy. You have a life outside the relationship and any reasonable man would understand that you need to give that aspect of your life the adequate attention it deserves. But if you begin to pretend that you are unavailable so that he will not think you are desperate, well guess what? You are showing desperation. If he calls you on phone, for example, and you deliberately refuse to answer even though you were not busy, why get excited over listening to his voicemail? If he texts you and you deliberately wait for hours to text him back, why obsessing over your response while waiting to text him back? You are simply setting yourself up to behave desperately and dishonestly. Your best bet is to find a healthy balance between other aspects of your life and your relationship. Be there for him if you are available.

3. **Waiting a specific amount of dates before having sex with him**: Time is not a good measure when it comes to having sex. Whether you meet a guy and have sex with him within a couple of hours or you waited four to five dates

before sleeping with him isn't really relevant. What matters is the quality of the time you shared, not the quantity or amount of time or dates you've been on together. In other words, why you have sex with a man is more important than when you have sex with him. Are you using sex to push him into commitment, or are you looking to have a more intimate connection with him? Does it feel right and natural or is it out of necessity? If you can answer these questions honestly, you will know when to have sex with a man you like.

4. **Pretending you are not interested in him**: Showing a man that you are interested in him doesn't push him away; instead, it draws him closer. Showing him that you are interested in him is what gets him intrigued in the first place. On the other hand, desperation or feeling that your self-worth depends on having a man in your life is what pushes men away. And the reason is simple. No man wants to feel he was chosen to fill a spot that any other man could have filled. He wants to feel that he earned the spot. Desperate women will accept just about any man that comes their way.

He's Now Your Man: The Rules are Now Different

Men are hunters by nature and they like to chase their game. Remove the chase from the hunt and the fun in hunting goes out the window. Give him the game on a platter of gold and he becomes bored. Once a man catches his game, the excitement of the chase is gone and he begins the search for another game to hunt down. Men are wired that way and for a good reason too. Without the chase, there would be a steady decline in birthing new offspring, and a gradual facing off of the human race. Don't hate them for being who they are; instead, use that knowledge to your advantage.

Once you've attracted a man and he's in a relationship with you, the rules have changed. Your focus is now on how to constantly give the sense of chasing you. This does not mean pleasing him at your own detriment. You must do what is mutually satisfying for both of you. Keeping a man doesn't mean you are his slave, rather, if you play your game right, your man will worship you. I have outlined a few important things that you can do to keep the chase alive in your relationship. Follow them, tweak them, and come up with great ideas to help keep the flame of your relationship burning.

Keeping the Flame Burning

The following tips can help you maintain a passionate relationship even after decades of being together with your man.

1. **Schedule weekend getaways**: It is surprising the number of couples who go on weekend getaways and get drawn in activities that they only have time for sex at night. First of all, the reason for going away for the weekend is to get away from activities. So, here's what I suggest you do. Check in to your hotel room, switch off your phone and put up the "do not disturb" sign. Next, shower and have sex. Have sex all through. That is how to enjoy a weekend getaway.

2. **Appreciate him and stroke his ego**: Compliment his achievement. Be genuinely proud of him and what he does. Make him feel like a capable man. Shower him with appreciation even for the little things he does, and he'll do more. Genuinely stroking his ego and appreciating him is meeting one of his core subconscious needs. A man will always go where he is acknowledged, appreciated, and made to feel like a true man.

3. **Shave him and allow him to shave you**: Offer to shave his face. This tells him you are into him

more than any words can. It doesn't matter whether you know how to shave him or not, and you don't even have to complete the shaving. Be playful about the process. Put some shaving cream on his nose and enjoy hearty laughter together. If you have established a lot of trust in your relationship, you can shave his pubic hair and also allow him to shave yours. He will always look forward to the shaving experience.

4. **Befriend his friends and wow them**: Trying to separate a man from his "gang" is not likely to put you in his "good" book. Unless he is a lone wolf, or his friends are beginning to get him into trouble, don't try to make enemies with them. Instead, become friends with those you think are a good influence on him. Men who are devoted to their friends are usually torn between their women and their friends. Instead of giving him a difficult time and making him choose between your and his friends, befriend them and you make life easier for him by mending the tear between home and friends. Also, if you make them think you are a great girl and a positive influence on him, he will cling to you more because he feels he has one of the best girls in his social circle.

5. **Play with him a lot**: Men find playful women very attractive. Give him an unexpected wink even in public places. Whisper crazy nothings into his ears, especially when people are around. He will look forward to being alone with you. Stick out your tongue and make playful faces at him. Sneak behind him and tickle him. When he seems engrossed in something touch his nose or gently pull his ears. Make the times you share together a memorable one that he looks forward to returning to.

6. **Have deep conversations**: Although this is not something sexy, men find a woman very attractive if she does participate in intellectual discussions and is interested in his personal development. Being sexy can attract a man, but if your conversations are usually shallow, lack any essence or tends to be focused only on romance, he may soon become tired because you don't offer him any intellectual stimulation. Nudge him toward achieving his goals and be passionate about reaching your own goals too. He will see you not only as a sex goddess but an intelligent partner he can depend on.

7. **Give him breathing space**: Men need their space. Remember in Chapter 2, I mentioned the

special empty compartment in a man's brain. Often, when a man is stressed he goes to the compartment containing absolutely nothing and remains there for as long as he needs to ease off the stress. Interrupting him when he needs to be alone will escalate his feeling of stress. If you notice that your man needs space, give him space. It tells him that you understand him and respect him enough not to bother him when he needs to be alone.

8. **Public display of affection**: While not all men will want to respond to a public display of affection, they still love it. When you kiss him, hug him tightly, fondle him, or cling onto his arms in public, you make him feel like your powerful and sexy hero.

9. **Put on his clothes**: Generally, a man finds it sexy to see his woman putting on his shirt with only her lingerie. To make it sexier, leave the buttons undone. The more casual you are in his shirt, the more turned on he becomes.

10. **Take initiative in bed**: Just because he is now your man doesn't mean you should stop taking charge during sex. Waiting for him to make the first move every night and allowing him to

constantly take the lead will make him start seeing sex with you as a chore. Dominate him in bed; it is part of showing how confident you are in yourself.

Conclusion

It's time to act. But don't just act; put the pedal to the metal! Don't just sit around in the hope that someday your ideal man or crush will finally come around to ask you out on a date. It hardly ever happens that way. The men that come your way may not be the type of men you truly want. Go out and get the man you truly desire. Remember that the patient dog has no option but to eat whatever bones are left; fattest or no fattest bone. The quickest dog, however, eats the fattest and most desirous steak.

Don't let limiting cultural or religious beliefs hold you back from experiencing true happiness in your life. We are designed to enjoy life. Take a good look at your feminine self and see how your intricate body is optimized for maximum pleasure. Don't let all that go to waste, especially in your youthful years. You can begin right now to break free from any ideology that tends to limit your sense of enjoyment. Life is meant to be fun!

You and I are not men, but we agree that men allow themselves to be who they are; they allow themselves to follow their natural hunter instincts. Why then should ours—women—be different? Flirting and seduction is part of our instincts. The man cannot hunt for you or chase after you if he doesn't even notice you, in the first place. The hunter sets his trap only in the places where he notices footprints of his kill. Tempt him, lure him, deliberately leave footprints to make him come looking for you. Quit sitting around and wasting away.

I have seen lots of smart, beautiful, strong, and intelligent women suffer in silence and cry out their eyes every night because they can't be with the man they want or because men only think of them as smart but not sexy enough to be with. Don't be that woman!

It may not be possible for you to use every technique outlined in this book. But you certainly must have found a few that completely resonated with you. Apply those even it if means taking baby steps. You will get better and better as you do so.

It is my burning desire to see more of us women liberate ourselves from the unnecessary timid attitude with which we approach dating and relationships. Living a happy and fulfilled life is actually easier than we have been led to believe. But it all starts with a shift in our attitudes. Life is fun. Flirting is fun. For the modern woman, flirting is life!

References

Bakos, S. C. (2008). *The sex bible for women*. Quiver, Quayside Publishing Group. ISBN-13: 978-1-59233-334-9

Riley, K. (1995). *Sexual secrets for men*. Random House Australia. ISBN-10: 0091831377

Greene, R. (2001). *The art of seduction*. Penguin Books; Reprint edition (October 7, 2003). ISBN-13: 978-0142001196

Sparks, N. (2015). *As you are*. Createspace Independent Publishing Platform. ISBN: 1517737893

Psychologies (2018). *How to master the art of flirting*. Retrieved October 6, 2019, from https://www.psychologies.co.uk/how-master-art-flirting

Fisher, H. (2016). *Anatomy of love: A natural history of mating, marriage and why we stray*. W. W. Norton & Company. Revised and Updated with a New Introduction edition (February 1, 2016) ISBN-13: 978-0393285222.

Bad Girls Bible (2013). *How flirt with a guy: 9 tips to make him uncontrollably attracted to you*. Retrieved October 13, 2019, from https://badgirlsbible.com/how-to-flirt-with-a-guy

www.ingramcontent.com/pod-product-compliance
Lightning Source LLC
Chambersburg PA
CBHW061808250726

48657CB00001B/336